The Complete
MRCS
Volume 2

System Modules

Edited by

Joseph K. C. Huang FRCS
Specialist Registrar in General Surgery
Anglia/Cambridge Region

Marc C. Winslet MS FRCS
Professor of Surgery and Head of Department
Royal Free Hospital and
University College Medical School
London

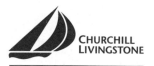
CHURCHILL
LIVINGSTONE

EDINBURGH   LONDON   NEW YORK   PHILADELPHIA   ST LOUIS   SYDNEY   TORONTO   2000

CHURCHILL LIVINGSTONE
An imprint of Harcourt Publishers Limited

© Harcourt Publishers Limited 2000

 is a registered trademark of Harcourt Publishers Limited

First published 2000

ISBN 0443 064571

British Library Cataloguing in Publication Data
A catalogue record for this book is available from the British Library

Library of Congress Cataloging in Publication Data
A catalog record for this book is available from the Library of Congress

Medical knowledge is constantly changing. As new information
becomes available, changes in treatment, procedures, equipment and
the use of drugs become necessary. The editors and the publishers have,
as far as it is possible, taken care to ensure that the information given in
this text is accurate and up to date. However, readers are strongly advised
to confirm that the information, especially with regard to drug usage,
complies with the latest legislation and standards of practice.

The
publisher's
policy is to use
paper manufactured
from sustainable forests

Printed by Bell & Bain Ltd., Glasgow

Preface

The aim of this book is to assist candidates in their final preparation for the MRCS examination, by allowing self-assessment of major parts of the syllabus, which will highlight areas of deficiency. It is not intended to be a comprehensive overview of the syllabus, which is already provided in the distance learning or STEP course published by the Royal College of Surgeons of England.

By their nature books containing MCQs cover certain areas in greater depth than others. It is not intended that the text should represent a substitute for extensive clinical reading, but rather act as a complement to it.

Each question includes a short answer section containing relevant background information and clinical comment where appropriate. Some of the answers will generate discussion and controversy reflecting normal clinical practice and hopefully stimulating further research and evaluation.

London, 2000

M. C. W.
J. K. C. H.

Contributors

Ajit Abraham MS FRCS
Specialist Registrar in General
Surgery, North-East Thames
Region, London
Questions and answers 5.21–5.56

Darryl Baker PhD FRCS (Gen)
Consultant Surgeon, Royal Free
Hospital, London
Questions and answers 2.1–2.40

Tim Briggs BSc MS FRCS Urol
Consultant Urologist, Barnet
General Hospital, London
Questions and answers 5.1–5.20

K. S. Cheng MA MB BChir FRCS
Specialist Registrar in General
Surgery, North-East Thames
Region, London
Questions and answers 2.1–2.40

Tim Davidson ChM MRCP FRCS
Consultant Surgeon, Royal Free
Hospital, London
Questions and answers 3.35–3.50

Oswald N. Fernando FRCS FRCS(E)
Consultant Transplant Surgeon,
Royal Free Hospital, London
Questions and answers 5.21–5.56

Nicholas Goddard MB FRCS
Consultant Orthopaedic Surgeon,
Royal Free Hospital, London
Questions and answers 1.1–1.62

Joseph K. C. Huang FRCS
Specialist Registrar in General
Surgery, Anglia/Cambridge
Region
Questions and answers 3.51–3.77

Frances Hughes MS FRCS
Surgical Registrar in General
Surgery, North-East Thames
Region, London
*Questions and answers 4.1–4.40,
4.81–4.83*

Frank Lee FRCS
Specialist Registrar in Urology,
North-East Thames Region,
London
Questions and answers 5.1–5.20

Yasser Mohsen MS FRCS (Gen)
Specialist Registrar in General
Surgery, North-East Thames
Region, London
Questions and answers 4.41–4.80

Robert E. Quiney BSc FRCS FRCSEd
Consultant ENT Surgeon, Royal
Free Hospital, London
Questions and answers 3.1–3.34

S. A. Wajed FRCS
Specialist Registrar, North-East
Thames Region, London;
Research Fellow, Department of
Surgery, University of Southern
California, USA
Questions and answers 3.35–3.50

Marc C. Winslet MS FRCS
Professor of Surgery and Head of
Department, Royal Free Hospital
and University College Medical
School, London
*Questions and answers
3.51–3.77, 4.1–4.40, 4.81–4.83*

Contents

Locomotor system

1.1 Rheumatoid arthritis is commonly associated with:
A. Morning stiffness.
B. Ulnar deviation of the fingers at the MCP joints.
C. Positive rheumatoid factor.
D. Flexor tendon ruptures.
E. Atlanto-axial instability.

1.2 Rheumatoid arthritis (RA) is commonly associated with:
A. Ulnar deviation at the PIP joints.
B. Minimal synovial hypertrophy.
C. Dorsal subluxation of the MCP joints.
D. A varus deformity at the knee.
E. Nodules on the flexor aspects of the limbs.

1.3 Rheumatoid arthritis:
A. Is a systemic disease.
B. Predominantly affects the synovium.
C. Mainly affects the IP joints of the hand.
D. May result in LMNL signs in the legs.
E. Does not usually result in deformity.

1.4 The following conditions are frequently associated with rheumatoid arthritis:
A. Macrocytic anaemia.
B. Splenomegaly.
C. Nail pitting.
D. Pericarditis.
E. Vasculitis.

1.5 The pathological features of rheumatoid arthritis include:
A. Synovial proliferation.
B. Enzyme production in the articular cartilage leading to chondrocyte destruction.
C. Ligament contractures.
D. Synovial fluid rich in proteolytic enzymes.
E. Frequent rupture of the finger flexor tendons.

1.6 Carpal tunnel syndrome is commonly associated with:
- **A.** Diabetes.
- **B.** Rheumatoid arthritis.
- **C.** Supracondylar fracture of the elbow.
- **D.** Thoracic outlet syndrome.
- **E.** Acromegaly.

1.7 Dupuytren's disease is characterized by:
- **A.** Thickening of the palmar aponeurosis.
- **B.** An autosomal dominant gene.
- **C.** Diabetes.
- **D.** An association with liver disease.
- **E.** A greater prevalence in women than in men.

1.8 Other associations with Dupuytren's disease include:
- **A.** Flexion contractures of the MCP/PIP joints.
- **B.** Rheumatoid arthritis.
- **C.** Gout.
- **D.** The use of vibrating tools.
- **E.** Raynaud's phenomenon.

1.9 The characteristic deformity in Dupuytren's disease is the result of contracture of:
- **A.** The deep flexor muscles of the hand.
- **B.** The skin of the palm.
- **C.** The palmaris longus muscle.
- **D.** The palmar aponeurosis.
- **E.** The intrinsic muscles of the hand.

1.10 The common late complications of total hip replacement are:
- **A.** Infection.
- **B.** Loosening.
- **C.** Dislocation.
- **D.** Deep venous thrombosis.
- **E.** Periprosthetic fracture.

1.11 In osteomalacia:
- **A.** The serum calcium is normal or low.
- **B.** The urinary calcium is low.
- **C.** Serum phosphate is high.
- **D.** Serum alkaline phosphatase is low.
- **E.** Bone biopsy shows inadequate mineralization.
- **F.** The technetium bone scan is normal.

1.12 The following statements concerning osteoporosis are correct:
  A. The composition of bone is normal but there is an insufficient amount.
  B. It is associated with long-term corticosteroid therapy.
  C. The radiographic features are of decreased bone density and thin cortices.
  D. It is commoner after the menopause in women.
  E. It is a common cause of vertebral fractures.
  F. It can be treated by administration of calcium/Vitamin D supplements.

1.13 When standing with the knees locked in full extension:
  A. The rectus femoris is contracted.
  B. The popliteus is contracted.
  C. The posterior capsule of the knee is tight.
  D. The anterior cruciate is lax.
  E. The femoral nerve is intact.

1.14 Congenital (developmental) dislocation of the hip:
  A. Is commoner in boys than girls.
  B. May only be apparent when the child starts to walk.
  C. Causes a delay in walking.
  D. Can usually be detected on routine neonatal screening.
  E. Is confirmed when the ossification centre of the femoral head appears late.
  F. Results in shortening of the leg.

1.15 A moderate sized acute disc protrusion at the L4/L5 level will result in:
  A. Loss of perianal sensation.
  B. Weakness of ankle dorsiflexion.
  C. Weakness of ankle plantar flexion.
  D. Weakness of extensor hallucis longus.
  E. A normal ankle reflex.
  F. A reduced knee reflex.
  G. Altered sensation on the lateral border of the foot.

1.16 Avascular necrosis of the head of the femur is associated with:
A. Gout.
B. Gaucher's disease.
C. Haemophilia.
D. Diabetes.
E. Deep-sea divers.
F. Long-term steroid therapy.

1.17 The characteristic radiological features of osteoarthritis include:
A. Periarticular osteoporosis.
B. Subchondral sclerosis.
C. Loss of joint space.
D. Erosions.
E. Osteophytes.
F. Cyst formation.
G. Soft-tissue swelling.

1.18 Primary hyperparathyroidism usually causes:
A. Raised serum calcium.
B. Raised alkaline phosphatase.
C. Raised serum phosphate.
D. Raised urinary calcium.

1.19 Primary hyperparathyroidism is characterized by:
A. Pathological fractures.
B. Peptic ulceration.
C. Muscle weakness.
D. Muscle tetany.
E. Low serum calcium.

1.20 The following are classical features of carpal tunnel syndrome:
A. Altered sensation over the medial fingers.
B. Nocturnal dysaesthesia.
C. Wasting of the first dorsal interosseus muscle.
D. Weakness of the abductor digiti minimi.
E. Nerve conduction studies are commonly normal in the early stages.

1.21 Haemophilia A:
  A. Is the result of an autosomal recessive inheritance pattern.
  B. Is caused by Factor IX deficiency.
  C. Most commonly affects the hip and shoulder joints.
  D. Results in a normal prothrombin time.
  E. Causes OA of the ankle.

1.22 Sickle-cell disease:
  A. Is the result of abnormal haemoglobin synthesis.
  B. Causes chronic anaemia.
  C. Is associated with avascular necrosis of the hip.
  D. Is associated with unusual infections.
  E. Responds well to steroid therapy.
  F. Unusually presents with bone pain.

1.23 The following are true concerning nerve injury:
  A. Neurapraxia has the best prognosis for recovery.
  B. Neurotmesis has the worst prognosis for recovery.
  C. Axonotmesis is the result of complete transection of the nerve.
  D. Nerves regenerate at the rate of approximately 1 cm a month.

1.24 The following act as internal rotators of the shoulder:
  A. Deltoid.
  B. Latissimus dorsi.
  C. Pectoralis minor.
  D. Serratus anterior.
  E. Infraspinatus.

1.25 Concerning the structure of normal articular (hyaline) cartilage:
  A. The framework consists of type I collagen fibres.
  B. The matrix is produced by chondrocytes.
  C. Damaged collagen fibres are repaired by fibroblasts.
  D. There is minimal water content.
  E. It relies on the synovial fluid for its nutrition.
  F. There is a rich blood supply arising from the subchondral bone.
  G. It contains many nerve fibres.

1.26 Technetium scanning may be helpful in the diagnosis of:
   A. Developmental dislocation of the hips.
   B. Osteoid osteoma.
   C. Fracture of the carpal scaphoid.
   D. Osteomalacia.
   E. Secondary malignant deposits in the brain.

1.27 Normal bone:
   A. Consists of bone lamellae surrounding a central canal containing osteoblasts and neurovascular bundles.
   B. Contains osteocytes which are involved in bone resorption and bone formation.
   C. Contains 40% collagen in the intercellular matrix.
   D. Has hydroxyapatite in the inorganic phase.
   E. Contains 20% water by weight.

1.28 The following statements concerning tuberculosis are correct:
   A. It is caused by a Gram-negative organism.
   B. In the UK, it is generally of the bovine type.
   C. Bone infection is a result of haematogenous spread.
   D. It affects synovial joints more frequently than the diaphysis of long bones.

1.29 The ulnar nerve supplies the following muscles:
   A. Abductor pollicis brevis.
   B. Adductor pollicis.
   C. Opponens pollicis.
   D. Abductor digiti minimi.
   E. Flexor pollicis longus.
   F. Flexor pollicis brevis.
   G. First dorsal interosseus.

1.30 Horner syndrome is characterized by:
   A. A dilated pupil.
   B. Ptosis.
   C. Exophthalmos.
   D. Loss of sweating over the forehead on the affected side.
   E. Weakness of the muscles supplied by the third cranial nerve.

1.31 With regard to the anatomical snuffbox:
- **A.** The abductor pollicis longus and extensor pollicis brevis tendons form one boundary.
- **B.** The abductor pollicis brevis tendon forms the dorsal boundary.
- **C.** The radial nerve can be palpated deep to the extensor pollicis longus tendon.
- **D.** The scaphoid forms the entirety of the floor.
- **E.** The princeps pollicis artery is palpable on the floor of the snuffbox.

1.32 In a tension pneumothorax:
- **A.** The trachea is central.
- **B.** The breath sounds are equal on both sides.
- **C.** The neck veins are distended.
- **D.** There is hyperresonance on percussion of the affected side.
- **E.** Immediate treatment is by insertion of a chest drain and underwater seal.

1.33 Mandatory radiographs of a severely injured patient include:
- **A.** The skull.
- **B.** The PA chest.
- **C.** The AP cervical spine.
- **D.** The AP pelvis.

1.34 A six-year-old child is brought into Accident and Emergency following a road traffic accident. The pulse is 120, BP is 70/40 and respiratory rate is 40. The following measures are appropriate:
- **A.** Set up an i.v. infusion and rapidly infuse 1000 ml of Hartmann's solution.
- **B.** Administer 24% oxygen by mask.
- **C.** Intubate the child.
- **D.** Perform a diagnostic peritoneal lavage.

1.35 The indications for an emergency chest drain include:
- **A.** An open chest wound.
- **B.** A haemothorax.
- **C.** Pericardial tamponade.
- **D.** Fractured ribs with a flail segment.
- **E.** Confirmed tension pneumothorax.

1.36 The following are potential reasons for a deteriorating condition after the institution of IPPV:
A. Reduced venous return and a secondary reduction in cardiac output.
B. A misplaced endotracheal tube.
C. Conversion of a simple pneumothorax into a tension pneumothorax.

1.37 The following statements are true concerning shock:
A. It is defined as inadequate tissue perfusion.
B. Treatment is aimed at restoring blood volume.
C. There is increased fluid sequestered in the third space.
D. Oxygen should be administered at 100%.

1.38 The signs of pericardial tamponade include:
A. Distended neck veins.
B. Widened pulse pressure.
C. Quiet heart sounds.
D. Gallop rhythm.
E. Reduced height of the R wave on ECG.
F. Pulsus paradoxus.
G. Normal blood pressure.

1.39 The following statements are characteristic of Class 2 hypovolaemic shock:
A. Blood loss is 30–40% .
B. Respiratory rate is 20–30.
C. There is normal capillary return.
D. Systolic blood pressure decreases.
E. Pulse pressure decreases.
F. Urinary output is > 30 ml/h.
G. The patient is confused.

1.40 Clinical features that might suggest pulmonary contusions include:
A. Blast exposure.
B. Chest wall tenderness.
C. Progressive hypoxia.
D. Haemoptysis.
E. Crepitation.

1.41 Emergency thoracotomy should be considered in the following situations:
  A. Immediate drainage from a chest tube of 1000 ml.
  B. Continued blood drainage of 200 ml/h.
  C. Signs of cardiac injury.
  D. Pericardial tamponade.
  E. Large open pneumothorax.

1.42 The following structures are likely to be injured following a pelvic fracture with disruption of the pelvic ring:
  A. Urethra.
  B. Prostate.
  C. Bladder.
  D. Major blood vessels.
  E. Neurological injury.

1.43 Urgent referral to a neurosurgical unit should be considered under the following circumstances:
  A. A deteriorating level of consciousness.
  B. Longitudinal parietal skull fracture.
  C. Focal neurological signs in the absence of a skull fracture.
  D. Disorientation persisting for more than 8 h.
  E. Persistent coma after adequate resuscitation.
  F. Open skull fracture.
  G. Depressed skull fracture.

1.44 The following results would suggest a positive result following diagnostic peritoneal lavage:
  A. >10 000 RBC/mm^3.
  B. >500 WBC/mm^3.
  C. Presence of faecal matter.
  D. Presence of a pneumoperitoneum.
  E. Presence of urine.

1.45 Fracture of the surgical neck humerus may be complicated by damage to:
  A. The radial nerve.
  B. The median nerve.
  C. The posterior cord of the brachial plexus
  D. The brachial artery.
  E. The axillary nerve.

1.46 Division of the radial nerve in the upper arm results in:
A. Wrist drop.
B. Weakness of the extensor carpi radialis longus.
C. Loss of active extension at the MCP joints.
D. Loss of active extension at the IP joints.
E. Weakness of opposition of the thumb.
F. Sensory loss over the dorsum of the first web space.
G. Wasting of the first dorsal interosseous muscle.

1.47 Supracondylar fractures of the humerus in children are often associated with:
A. Damage to the radial nerve.
B. Damage to the median nerve.
C. Damage to the ulnar nerve.
D. Damage to the brachial artery.
E. Damage to the musculocutaneous nerve.
F. Volkmann's ischaemic contracture.

1.48 In a Colles' fracture:
A. The distal fragment is displaced posteriorly.
B. The distal fragment is displaced laterally.
C. The distal fragment is displaced anteriorly.
D. The distal fragment is displaced medially.
E. The ulna is intact.

1.49 The common complications of a Colles' fracture include:
A. Malunion.
B. Non-union.
C. Carpal tunnel syndrome.
D. Reflex sympathetic dystrophy (Sudeks atrophy).
E. Rupture of the tendon of extensor pollicis brevis.

1.50 Concerning fracture of the scaphoid:
A. It is the most frequently fractured of the carpal bones.
B. Avascular necrosis of the distal pole is common.
C. Non-union occurs in approximately 10% of cases.
D. The major blood supply enters from the proximal pole.
E. Displaced fractures of the wrist should be immobilized in plaster.

1.51 Concerning fractures of the neck of the femur:
   A. A displaced extracapsular fracture should be fixed with a DHS (pin and plate).
   B. A displaced extracapsular fracture should be treated by hemiarthroplasty.
   C. An undisplaced intracapsular fracture should be fixed by screws.
   D. A displaced intracapsular fracture in a 40-year-old should be treated by hemiarthroplasty.
   E. A displaced intracapsular fracture in an 80-year-old should be treated by hemiarthroplasty.

1.52 Concerning compartment syndrome in the leg:
   A. It is invariably secondary to a fracture.
   B. The lateral compartment is most commonly affected.
   C. There is pain on passive plantar flexion of the toes.
   D. There is loss of sensation over the dorsum of the foot.
   E. The dorsalis pedis pulse is generally absent.
   F. It is confirmed by a compartment pressure measurement of 20 mmHg.

1.53 A ruptured anterior cruciate ligament has the following characteristics:
   A. It is usually accompanied by a 'crack' heard and felt in the knee at the moment of injury.
   B. It results in a slow onset effusion.
   C. The tibia sags posteriorly when viewed from the side.
   D. Lachmann's test is negative.
   E. A posterior draw test is positive.
   F. It is often associated with medial collateral ligament/medial meniscus lesions.

1.54 The following patterns of tibial shaft fractures are inherently unstable:
   A. Transverse.
   B. Oblique.
   C. Spiral.
   D. Comminuted.
   E. Butterfly.
   F. Open.

1.55 Fractures of the midshaft of the clavicle:
  A. Commonly do not unite.
  B. Should be treated by open reduction and internal fixation (ORIF) if they are displaced.
  C. May be complicated by damage to the cords of the brachial plexus.
  D. May be complicated by damage to the axillary artery.
  E. Generally unite within six weeks in an adult.

1.56 The following muscles are flexors of the wrist:
  A. Brachioradialis.
  B. Flexor carpi ulnaris.
  D. Pronator teres.
  E. Flexor digitorum profundus.
  F. Flexor pollicis brevis.

1.57 An anterolateral approach to the hip:
  A. Requires that the gluteal fascia be split.
  B. Passes anterior to gluteus medius.
  C. Passes anterior to tensor fascia lata.
  D. Passes anterior to rectus femoris.
  E. Is less likely to damage the sciatic nerve than with the posterolateral approach.

1.58 Concerning the posterolateral approach to the hip:
  A. The sciatic nerve passes superficial to the piriformis.
  B. The obturator externus is cut to expose the capsule.
  C. The hip is dislocated by internal rotation and flexion.
  D. The sciatic nerve is protected by retracting the gluteus minimus across it.
  E. Foot drop/weakness of dorsiflexion are the commonest neurological complications.

1.59 A 75-year-old patient presents with a shortened externally rotated leg. The following are likely causes:
  A. Extracapsular fracture of the neck of femur.
  B. Fracture of the femoral shaft.
  C. Posterior dislocation of the hip.
  D. Garden grade II fractured neck of femur.
  E. Fractured superior and inferior pubic rami.

1.60 Theme: Fracture management

Options:
A. Plaster of paris
B. Skeletal traction
C. External fixation
D. Internal fixation by plate and screws
E. Internal fixation by intramedullary nail

For each of the patients described below, select the single most appropriate management from the list of options above. Each option may be used once, more than once or not at all.

1. An 18-year-old man is injured during a motorcycle accident, and sustains head injuries, chest injuries and a fracture of the femoral shaft. His initial resuscitation includes intubation and ventilation. The fracture is a closed transverse fracture of the midshaft with minimal displacement following application of skin traction. What will be your definitive management of this fracture?

2. A 22-year-old motorcyclist sustains an isolated lower limb injury. He has sustained a minimally compound fracture of the midshaft of the tibia and fibula. The tibial fracture is transverse and there is a small wound, approximately 1 cm, overlying. What will be your definitive fracture management?

3. A 45-year-old woman has jumped from a considerable height sustaining a complex and comminuted distal tibial fracture (pilon fracture). There is considerable disruption of the distal tibial articular surface with the talus driven into the fracture splaying the fragments apart. What will be your initial fracture management?

1.61 Theme: Wound management

Options:
A. Primary closure
B. Healing by second intention
C. Delayed primary closure
D. Skin grafting
E. Application of flap

For each of the patients described below, select the single most appropriate management from the list of options above. Each option may be used once, more than once or not at all.

1. A 19-year-old has sustained a degloving type injury of the dorsum of the foot. He has lost an extensive area of skin and subcutaneous tissue leaving muscle and tendon sheaths exposed. There is no bony injury and no evidence of neurovascular compromise. How will you best achieve wound healing?

2. A 25-year-old man has sustained a partial amputation of his fingertip, losing approximately 1 cm^2 of skin, pulp and part of distal phalanx. He has not however lost any of the nail bed elements. How should the wound be managed?

3. A 22-year-old motorcyclist has sustained an open fracture of the distal tibia which is suitable for intramedullary nailing with distal locking screws. There is however a large soft tissue defect which will require coverage. What is the ideal way to manage this wound?

1.62 Theme: Head injuries

Options:
A. Concussion
B. Diffuse axonal injury
C. Extradural haematoma
D. Subdural haematoma
E. Open skull fracture

For each of the patients described below, select the single most appropriate diagnosis from the list of options above. Each option may be used once, more than once or not at all.

1. A 24-year-old man is brought to the emergency department in a deep coma following an assault. His GCS is 4 and was also recorded as being 4 at the scene. He displays bilateral symmetrical decerebrate extensor posturing to painful stimulus. His pupils are dilated and unreactive to light. There is no cardiorespiratory abnormality and he smells strongly of alcohol. What is the likely diagnosis?

2. A 36-year-old woman is injured in an RTA. At the scene she is witnessed as verbalizing, though confused. In the emergency department she is found to be deeply comatose, with a GCS of 5, now demonstrating decorticate flexion to painful stimuli, and not verbalizing. There is slight asymmetry of pupil size but both are reactive. What is the likely diagnosis?

Vascular system

2.1 Carotid stenosis:
A. May present with contralateral amaurosis fugax.
B. May present with homonymous hemianopia.
C. May present with hemisensory and or hemimotor signs.
D. May present with dysarthria and gait problems.
E. Should be treated by carotid endarterectomy in symptomatic patients.

2.2 Percutaneous transluminal angioplasty (PTA):
A. Has a primary patency rate of 40% at two years for superficial femoral artery angioplasty.
B. Is ideal for treating long stenosis of the superficial femoral artery with a long balloon.
C. Causes a higher bleeding complication rate than angiography.
D. Can cause dissection of the artery.
E. Can cause arterial thrombosis.

2.3 Occlusive aortoiliac disease:
A. Can present with Lhermitte's sign.
B. Can be treated by percutaneous transluminal angioplasty (PTA).
C. Has a patency rate of 95% at five years if treated by femoro-femoral bypass graft in unilateral disease.
D. Can present with isolated digital gangrene.

2.4 Differential diagnoses of lower leg ulcer include the following:
A. Acute pancreatitis.
B. Hyperparathyroidism.
C. Thyrotoxicosis.
D. Renal failure.
E. Ulcerative colitis.

2.5 Venous ulcers:
   A. Are typically painful.
   B. Occur predominantly in the gaiter area.
   C. Can occur in the absence of varicose veins.
   D. May show features of lymphoedema.
   E. May undergo malignant transformation.

2.6 Patients with the following conditions have higher risks of developing adverse reactions following angiography:
   A. Asthma.
   B. Liver failure.
   C. Heart failure.
   D. Renal failure.
   E. Diabetes mellitus treated with metformin.

2.7 The following conditions are associated with an increased risk of developing abdominal aortic aneurysm (AAA):
   A. Marfan syndrome.
   B. Alpha-1 antitrypsin deficiency.
   C. Ehlers–Danlos syndrome.
   D. Diabetes mellitus.
   E. Syphilis.

2.8 Lymphoedema:
   A. Commonly presents with ankle ulceration.
   B. Of the primary type commonly affects females.
   C. Is associated with recurrent Staphylococcus infection.
   D. Has a genetic association.
   E. Can present at a late age.

2.9 The following conditions are associated with Raynaud's phenomenon:
   A. Systemic lupus erythematosis (SLE).
   B. Hypothyroidism.
   C. Cryoglobulinaemia.
   D. Carcinoma of the bronchus.
   E. Systemic sclerosis.

2.10 Concerning aneurysms:
A. The blood is forced through a tear in the aortic media in a dissecting aneurysm.
B. Charcot–Bouchard aneurysms are associated with diabetic vascular disease.
C. Mycotic aneurysms are associated with malignant disease.
D. Aneurysms secondary to syphilis usually occur in the thoracic aorta.
E. Mortality from a dissecting aneurysm is 5% at 48 h.

2.11 Diabetics with peripheral vascular disease:
A. May present with painless ischaemic ulcers.
B. Should stop insulin treatment prior to angiography.
C. Account for 15% of amputations.
D. May have ankle brachial pressure index of or greater than one even in the presence of severe ischaemia.
E. Should have a good control of the blood sugar level to lower the risk of future limb amputation.

2.12 Raynaud's phenomenon:
A. Has an association with the oral contraceptive pill.
B. Can lead to gangrene of the digit.
C. Has been reported as a side effect of beta adrenoceptor antagonists.
D. Can be relieved by intra-arterial reserpine infusion during an acute attack.
E. Most commonly affects elderly men.

2.13 Giant cell arteritis:
A. Is associated with erythema nodosum.
B. Can present with sudden loss of vision in one eye.
C. Can present with jaw pain during mastication.
D. Is associated with polymyalgia rheumatica in over 80% of cases.
E. Can be confirmed by temporal artery biopsy in all cases.

2.14 Buerger's disease (thromboangiitis obliterans):
A. Is associated with HLA-A9 and HLA-B5 genes.
B. Affects women more than men.
C. Has a strong association with cigarette smoking.
D. Causes gangrene in the lower limb only.
E. Can affect nerves and veins.

2.15 Tumours of the blood vessels include:
  A. Glomus tumour of the nail bed.
  B. Granulosa cell tumour.
  C. Kaposi's sarcoma.
  D. Hamartomata.
  E. Cholangiocarcinoma.

2.16 In the 'subclavian steal' syndrome:
  A. There is occlusion of the vertebral artery.
  B. There is occlusion of the carotid artery.
  C. The cause can be a cervical rib.
  D. The patient may present with dizziness.
  E. The patient may present with amaurosis fugax.

2.17 Tetralogy of Fallot consists of:
  A. Atrial septal defect.
  B. Left to right shunt.
  C. Right ventricular hypertrophy.
  D. Pulmonary stenosis.
  E. Overriding of the root of aorta to the left side of the heart.

2.18 Early (that is, less than 30 days) causes of vein graft failure include:
  A. Atherosclerosis.
  B. Inadequate run-off.
  C. Neointimal hyperplasia.
  D. Graft thrombosis.
  E. Aneurysmal deterioration of graft.

2.19 Vascular synthetic graft infection presents with:
  A. Pyrexia of unknown origin and malaise.
  B. Melaena.
  C. Wound sinus.
  D. False aneurysm.
  E. Graft thrombosis.

2.20 The following statements concerning aneurysmal dilatation of vascular grafts are correct:
A. It can affect vein graft.
B. Infection is a recognized cause.
C. Deterioration of a Dacron graft is a recognized cause.
D. The commonest site is at the femoral anastomosis of aorto-femoral and femoro-popliteal grafts.
E. It should be treated conservatively.

2.21 In disruption of the thoracic aorta in a patient from an RTA:
A. The mechanism of injury is almost always from rapid acceleration force.
B. The site of disruption is usually at the level of the ascending aorta.
C. The majority of patients will reach the hospital alive.
D. Suspicion is increased with widening of the mediastinum on CXR.
E. Suspicion is increased with the presence of left apical cap on CXR.

2.22 Thrombolysis is contraindicated in the following clinical situations:
A. Myocardial infarction within two weeks.
B. Infected graft.
C. Cerebrovascular accident greater than six months.
D. Pulmonary embolism within two weeks.
E. Vascular surgery within two weeks.

2.23 The following clinical features are associated with Klippel–Trenaunay syndrome:
A. Varicose veins.
B. Limb shortage.
C. Limb gigantism.
D. Haemangiomas.
E. Digital abnormality.

2.24 Takayasu's arteritis:
A. Affects medium and small muscular arteries.
B. Predominantly affects females.
C. Predominantly affects elderly patients.
D. Is mainly diagnosed by angiography.
E. Is characterized by a grossly elevated ESR.

2.25 An abdominal aortic aneurysm (AAA):
   A. Can present with frank haematuria.
   B. Has a mortality rate from elective surgery of about 1%.
   C. Is characterized by impotence as a significant complication of surgery.
   D. Lists ischaemic bowel as a recognized complication of surgery.
   E. Is associated with aneurysm elsewhere.

2.26 In endoluminal aortic aneurysm repair:
   A. The morphology of the aneurysm is not important.
   B. Femoro-femoral crossover graft is indicated with some types of stent.
   C. Perigraft leakage is a complication specific to endoluminal repair.
   D. Distant embolization does not occur.
   E. The procedure is performed under local anaesthetic.

2.27 The following clinical features are associated with Leriche syndrome:
   A. Absent femoral pulses.
   B. Bilateral buttock claudication.
   C. Carotid stenosis.
   D. Abdominal aortic aneurysm.
   E. Impotence.

2.28 Woven Dacron graft has the following characteristics compared with knitted Dacron graft:
   A. Higher porosity.
   B. Higher risk of aneurysmal dilatation.
   C. It is flexible in any direction.
   D. Greater compliance.
   E. A tendency to fray at the edges.

2.29 The following are characteristic of the feet of diabetic patients:
   A. Gangrene occurs even in the presence of palpable foot pulses.
   B. Ulcers are usually painless.
   C. Ulcers usually occur around the gaiter area.
   D. High Doppler foot pressures exclude arterial disease.
   E. Blood glucose level is the most important prognostic factor in diabetic foot.

2.30 **The following are risk factors associated with varicose veins:**
- **A.** Trauma.
- **B.** Pregnancy.
- **C.** Deep vein thrombosis.
- **D.** Leriche syndrome.
- **E.** Klippel–Trenaunay syndrome.

2.31 **During varicose vein surgery:**
- **A.** The femoral vein lies lateral to the femoral artery.
- **B.** The saphenopopliteal junction is always found at the level of the proximal transverse popliteal crease.
- **C.** Perforator incompetence can be dealt with by SEPS.
- **D.** The Trendelenberg procedure is indicated for saphenopopliteal incompetence.
- **E.** Stripping of the long saphenous vein to the ankle increases the risk of nerve damage.

2.32 **The following statements are true of cervical sympathectomy:**
- **A.** It is useful in the treatment of reflex sympathetic dystrophy.
- **B.** It is useful in the treatment of palmar hyperhydrosis.
- **C.** Horner syndrome is not a recognized complication.
- **D.** Compensatory hyperhydrosis is a recognized complication.
- **E.** Frey syndrome is a recognized complication.

2.33 **Expanded polytetrafluoroethylene (ePTFE) grafts in clinical use have the following characteristics:**
- **A.** A higher risk of aneurysmal dilatation.
- **B.** They are impervious to blood.
- **C.** They are electronegative.
- **D.** They are hydrophobic.
- **E.** They are chemically inert.

2.34 **The following vasculitic conditions primarily affect the aorta:**
- **A.** Rheumatoid arthritis.
- **B.** Wegener's granulomatosis.
- **C.** Polyarteritis nodosa.
- **D.** Takayasu's arteritis.
- **E.** Allergic vasculitis.

2.35 Hypersplenism:
   A. Can be caused by rheumatoid arthritis.
   B. Can be caused by lymphoma.
   C. Results in thrombocytosis.
   D. Results in leucopenia.
   E. Results in thrombocytopenia.

2.36 Theme: Vascular surgical procedures

Options:
   A. Endarterectomy
   B. Sympathectomy
   C. Percutaneous transluminal angioplasty
   D. Femoro-popliteal bypass
   E. Axillo-bifemoral bypass
   F. Femoro-femoral bypass
   G. Aorto-bifemoral bypass

For each of the patients described below, select the single most appropriate procedure from the list of options above. Each option may be used once, more than once or not at all.

1. A patient with an infected aortic graft.

2. A patient with aortoiliac occlusion.

3. A patient with symptomatic carotid stenosis.

4. A patient undergoing endovascular repair of abdominal aortic aneurysm (AAA) with single lumen aortoiliac graft.

2.37 Theme: Vascular investigations (I)

Options:
A. Intra-arterial digital subtraction angiography
B. Intravenous digital angiography
C. Resting and post exercise doppler pressures
D. Duplex scan
E. Plethysmography
F. Venography
G. CT scan
H. Ultrasound scan

For each of the patients described below, select the single most appropriate investigation from the list of options above. Each option may be used once, more than once or not at all.

1. Assessment of the underlying cause in a patient with a cerebrovascular accident (CVA).

2. A patient with Leriche syndrome.

3. A patient with swollen painful calf.

4. Assessment of a patient with abdominal aortic aneurysm (AAA).

5. Assessment of a patient with calf pain on walking and palpable pulses.

2.38 Theme: Vascular investigations (II)

Options:
A. Arteriogram
B. Duplex doppler scan
C. Magnetic resonance imaging (MRI)
D. Ultrasound scan
E. Computer tomography scan (CT)
F. Venogram

For each of the patients described below, select the single most appropriate investigation from the list of options above. Each option may be used once, more than once or not at all.

1. Which is the investigation of choice for arterial graft surveillance?

2. Which gives the best measurement of the size of an abdominal aortic aneurysm?

3. Which is the investigation of choice for recurrent varicose veins?

4. Which is the work-up investigation for endoluminal aortic aneurysm surgery?

5. Which investigation can be used for patients with peripheral vascular disease, who have severe iodine allergy?

2.39 Theme: Leg ulcers

Options:
A. Diabetic
B. Arterial
C. Venous
D. Traumatic
E. Pyoderma gangrenosum
F. Pyogenic granuloma

For each of the descriptions below, select the single most likely condition referred to from the list of options above. Each option may be used once, more than once or not at all.

1. Graduated compression treatment is contraindicated.

2. Accounts for 80% of leg ulceration.

3. Has an association with inflammatory bowel disease.

4. Usually has a neuroischaemic origin.

5. Usually occurs around the gaiter area.

2.40 Theme: Causes and associations

Options:
A. Lipodermatosclerosis
B. Panniculitis
C. Pretibial myxoedema
D. Erythema nodosum
E. Erythema induratum
F. Thrombophlebitis migrans

For each of the questions below, select the single most likely diagnosis from the list of options above. Each option may be used once, more than once or not at all.

1. Which is caused by chronic venous insufficiency?

2. Which has an association with pancreatic carcinoma?

3. Which is caused by acute pancreatitis?

4. Which is associated with thyrotoxicosis?

5. Which has an association with inflammatory bowel disease?

27

Head and neck, endocrine system, and paediatric disorders

HEAD AND NECK

3.1 Laryngeal tumours:
   A. Most commonly arise in the subglottis.
   B. Are commonly caused by asbestos exposure.
   C. Commonly metastasize.
   D. Commonly present with stridor.
   E. Involvement of the recurrent laryngeal nerve is indicated by vocal cord palsy.

3.2 Benign paroxysmal vertigo:
   A. Is associated with head injury.
   B. Is caused by loose particles in the lateral semicircular canal.
   C. May require surgery.
   D. Should be managed with prochloperazine (Stemetil).
   E. Is not helped by Cawthorne–Cooksey exercises.

3.3 Otitis media with effusion:
   A. In children is associated with parental smoking.
   B. Is always associated with a conductive hearing loss.
   C. Can cause the eardrum to appear blue.
   D. Is best treated by early surgery.
   E. Causes facial weakness if left untreated.

3.4 Following nasal trauma:
   A. Leakage of cerebrospinal fluid is a common sequela.
   B. X-ray of the nasal bones is recommended.
   C. Manipulation of the nasal bones can be done easily up to six weeks afterwards.
   D. Septal haematoma is a common consequence.
   E. Epistaxis is treated with cautery.

3.5 Nasal polyps are associated with:
   A. Atopic asthma.
   B. Cystic fibrosis.
   C. Aspirin sensitivity.
   D. Allergic fungal sinusitis.
   E. Chronic infective sinusitis.

3.6 Complications of oroantral fistulae include:
   A. Facial numbness.
   B. Sinusitis.
   C. Nasal regurgitation of fluids.
   D. Anosmia.
   E. Hypernasal speech.

3.7 Following skullbase fracture of the temporal bone:
   A. CSF otorrhoea requires urgent surgical intervention.
   B. Facial palsy is usual.
   C. Haemotympanum is consistent with a conductive hearing loss.
   D. Fast phase nystagmus to the opposite ear is a good prognosis.
   E. Battle's sign confirms the diagnosis.

3.8 Lateral rhinotomy is used to excise:
   A. Inverted papilloma.
   B. Nasal polyps.
   C. Juvenile angiofibroma.
   D. Adenoids.
   E. Olfactory neuroblastoma.

3.9 Complications of grommet insertion include:
   A. Otorrhoea.
   B. Dizziness.
   C. Ear drum perforation.
   D. Tympanosclerosis.
   E. The development of retraction pockets.

3.10 Objective tinnitus can be caused by:
    A. Presbyacusis.
    B. Glomus jugulare tumour.
    C. Spasms of the tensor tympani muscle.
    D. Loud rock music.
    E. Ototoxic drugs such as gentamicin.

3.11 Regarding genetically based sensorineural deafness:
    A. Pendred syndrome usually causes hypothyroidism.
    B. In Usher syndrome the cochlea cells are abnormal.
    C. Aminoglycoside deafness may be caused by a mitochondrial DNA mutation.
    D. Profound sensorineural deafness is usually autosomal dominant.
    E. Radiology of the cochlea is abnormal.

3.12 Anosmia is caused by:
    A. Nasal polyps.
    B. Laryngectomy.
    C. Glue sniffing.
    D. Epstein–Barr virus.
    E. Sinusitis.

3.13 Ménière's disease (or syndrome) causes the following:
    A. High frequency fluctuating sensorineural deafness.
    B. Pulsatile tinnitus.
    C. Dizziness lasting for 20–60 s.
    D. Pressure in the affected ear.
    E. Otalgia.

3.14 Pharyngeal pouch:
    A. Often presents with hoarseness.
    B. Is premalignant.
    C. Is associated with gastro-oesophageal reflux.
    D. Is best surgically excised if small.
    E. Is congenital in origin.

3.15 The following are axial pattern flaps:
    A. Abbe–Esslander.
    B. Deltopectoral.
    C. Pectoralis major.
    D. Nasolabial.
    E. Tongue.

3.16 Regarding tracheostomy:
A. A common complication is vocal cord palsy.
B. Subglottic stenosis is more common in children.
C. Surgical emphysema is a frequent complication.
D. Horizontal incision of cartilage is preferable in children.
E. Indications include severe respiratory distress.

3.17 The following statements concerning carcinoma of the larynx are correct:
A. T1 and T2 have a high cure rate with radiotherapy.
B. T3 includes decreased mobility of the vocal cord.
C. Collar incision includes the tracheostomy stoma in the wound.
D. Salivary fistula is a common complication of surgery.
E. T3 N0 should have prophylactic neck dissection as part of the treatment.

3.18 A deviated nasal septum:
A. Is rarely congenital in origin.
B. Should always be managed by septoplasty and not submucosal resection.
C. Can cause snoring.
D. Is a common cause of sinusitis.
E. Always causes nasal obstruction.

3.19 Conductive hearing loss is caused by:
A. Syphilis.
B. Otosclerosis.
C. Otitis externa.
D. Tympanosclerosis.
E. Aminoglycoside antibiotics.

3.20 The following statements concerning topical steroid nasal sprays are correct:
A. They should not be used long term.
B. Long-term use causes rhinitis medicamentosa.
C. A significant part of their action occurs after systemic absorption.
D. They should be used in the head down and forward position.
E. They have no role in the management of rhinitis in children.

3.21 The following statements concerning facial palsy are correct:
- **A.** Neurotnmesis has a better prognosis than neuropraxia.
- **B.** Upper motor neurone lesions causes paralysis of occipitofrontalis.
- **C.** Electromyography is not useful in the first three days.
- **D.** Parotid malignancy causing palsy affects Schirmer's test.
- **E.** Vesicles in the ear suggest Ramsay–Hunt syndrome.

3.22 Otitis externa:
- **A.** Is usually painful.
- **B.** Is usually fungal.
- **C.** Is mainly treated by aural toilet.
- **D.** Often metastasizes if malignant.
- **E.** Causes cholesteatoma if untreated.

3.23 In thyroidectomy:
- **A.** The left recurrent laryngeal nerve is anterior to the inferior thyroid artery.
- **B.** Retrosternal extension usually requires thoracotomy.
- **C.** The superior laryngeal nerve can be damaged dividing the superior pedicle.
- **D.** Thyrotoxic crisis can be prevented with beta-blockers.
- **E.** Methylene blue helps define the parathyroids.

3.24 Otitis media with effusion:
- **A.** Causes permanent deafness.
- **B.** Is more common in adults.
- **C.** Presents with aural discharge.
- **D.** Rhinne's test is usually bone better than air conduction.
- **E.** Cholesteatoma is a frequent complication.

3.25 Indications for tonsillectomy include:
- **A.** Drooling.
- **B.** Recurrent tonsillitis.
- **C.** Sleep apnoea.
- **D.** Cleft palate.
- **E.** As part of an approach to the parapharyngeal space.

3.26 Ludwig's angina:
A. Is a consequence of dental sepsis.
B. Is caused by anaerobic bacteria in 20% of cases.
C. Can lead to respiratory distress.
D. Can be helpfully investigated by ultrasound scan.
E. Can be treated with oral antibiotics.

3.27 Nasal polyps:
A. Usually arise from the maxillary sinus.
B. Normally occur in atopic patients.
C. Are usually seen medial to the middle turbinate.
D. Should always be excised if they are unilateral.
E. Should be treated long-term with topical steroid drops.

3.28 Ear perforations:
A. Are deemed safe if marginal.
B. Should always be treated surgically.
C. Should not be managed by topical antibiotic ear drops.
D. Present with a greater hearing loss with anterior perforations than with posterior perforations.
E. The Weber test lateralizes to the normal opposite ear.

3.29 The following are true of snoring patients:
A. They can present with day-time hypersomnolence.
B. Epworth scores are useful in predicting obstructive sleep apnoea.
C. Palatal surgery may interfere with long-term use of nasal CPAP.
D. The snoring is most commonly caused by hypopharyngeal collapse.
E. A diagnosis of hyperthyroidism should be considered.

3.30 Branchial cysts:
A. Tend to occur in the elderly.
B. Are usually bilateral.
C. Present posterior to the sternomastoid muscle.
D. Are premalignant.
E. Are associated with tracks passing between the carotid bifurcation.

3.31 Causes of oroantral fistula include:
A. Maxillary carcinoma.
B. Penetrating injury.
C. Intranasal antrostomy.
D. Post-surgical ligation of the internal maxillary artery.
E. Dental extraction.

3.32 The following are first branchial arch derivatives:
A. Malleus.
B. Stapes.
C. Styloid process.
D. Mandible.
E. Thyroid gland.

3.33 The following ENT conditions are usually caused by single gene abnormalities:
A. Goldenhar syndrome.
B. Treacher–Collins syndrome.
C. Usher syndrome.
D. CHARGE association.
E. Osler's disease (haemorragic telangectasia).

3.34 Bell's palsy is caused by:
A. Forceps delivery.
B. Acoustic neuroma.
C. Cholesteatoma.
D. Tuberculosis.
E. Skullbase fracture.

ENDOCRINE SYSTEM

3.35 The thyroid gland:
A. Is derived from the first and second pharyngeal pouches.
B. Isthmus overlies the 5th and 6th tracheal rings normally.
C. Embryologically descends along the thyroglossal tract.
D. Is supplied by the superior thyroid artery branch of the internal carotid artery.
E. Is supplied by the inferior thyroid artery branch of the external carotid artery.

3.36 Thyroxine (T4):
A. Is formed from the iodination of tri-iodothyronine (T3).
B. Is bound to thyroglobulin in plasma serum.
C. Is converted to T3 at the tissues.
D. Increases carbohydrate absorption from the intestine.
E. Lowers oxygen consumption in the tissues.

3.37 A nodule in the thyroid gland:
A. May be a presentation of multinodular goitre.
B. Is unlikely to be a cyst if painful.
C. Should not be investigated with needle cytology.
D. Always requires excision.
E. Will require clinical examination to distinguish between a benign and a malignant nodule.

3.38 Thyroglossal cyst:
A. Is a midline swelling.
B. Results from the ultimo-branchial body embryologically.
C. May present as a papillary carcinoma.
D. Occurs only between the foramen caecum and the hyoid bone.
E. Is usually successfully treated by simple excision of the cyst.

3.39 Thyrotoxicosis:
A. Is the usual sequela of Hashimoto's disease.
B. Increases vascularity of the thyroid gland.
C. In Graves' disease is the result of excess pituitary TSH.
D. May cause cardiac arrythmias.
E. Can be caused by a solitary 'cold' nodule.

3.40 Regarding the recurrent laryngeal nerve:
A. It should be sought initially below the inferior thyroid artery.
B. It passess obliquely upwards and forwards.
C. It originates from the phrenic nerve in the thorax.
D. It supplies the cricopharyngeus muscle.
E. Complete unilateral palsy of this nerve results in hoarseness of the voice.

3.41 The adrenal glands:
A. Drain directly into the renal veins.
B. Secrete catecholamines from the zona glomerulosa.
C. Secrete aldosterone which enhances sodium retention.
D. Are sensitive to serum ACTH.
E. Respond to parasympathetic stimulation.

3.42 Phaechromocytoma:
A. Represent tumours of sympathetic neurones.
B. Are associated with the MEN I syndrome
C. May be found at the aortic bifurcation.
D. Are frequently bilateral.
E. Show familial tendency.

3.43 Cushing syndrome:
A. Is diagnosed by high serum ACTH.
B. Often presents with diabetes.
C. Can be caused by posterior pituitary tumours.
D. Results in increased urinary secretion of VMA.
E. Can be controlled with carbimazole.

3.44 Parathormone (PTH):
A. Is a peptide hormone.
B. Increases urinary phosphate excretion.
C. Requires Vitamin D as a precursor.
D. Serum levels are raised in chronic renal failure.
E. Stimulates osteoblastic activity.

3.45 Hyperparathyroidism:
- **A.** Is associated with MEN I syndrome.
- **B.** Can cause hypertension.
- **C.** Is commonly related to multiple parathyroid adenomata.
- **D.** Causes bone cyst formation.
- **E.** Is associated with pancreatitis.

3.46 Carcinoid tumours:
- **A.** Produce serotonin.
- **B.** Arise from anywhere in the gastrointestinal tract.
- **C.** Of the appendix frequently metastasize to the liver.
- **D.** Can be detected by levels of VMA in the urine.
- **E.** Originate from amine precursor uptake decarboxylase cells.

3.47 The following statements are true of multiple endocrine neoplasia (MEN):
- **A.** It originates from amine precursor uptake decarboxylase cells.
- **B.** Type I can present with hypoglycaemia.
- **C.** Type I can present with peptic ulceration.
- **D.** It shows familial tendency.
- **E.** Type IIA is associated with multiple neuroma.

3.48 Causes of hypercalcaemia include:
- **A.** Multiple myeloma.
- **B.** Chronic respiratory failure.
- **C.** Medullary carcinoma of the thyroid.
- **D.** Sarcoidosis.
- **E.** Bronchial carcinoma.

3.49 Cancers that commonly metastasize to bone include:
- **A.** Bronchial.
- **B.** Prostate.
- **C.** Ovarian.
- **D.** Testicular.
- **E.** Breast.

3.50 Theme: Thyroid neoplasia

Options:
A. Adenoma
B. Papillary
C. Follicular
D. Medullary
E. Anaplastic
F. Lymphoma

For each of the descriptions below, select the single most likely diagnosis from the list of options above. Each option may be used once, more than once or not at all.

1. Commonly spreads to lymph nodes.

2. Originates from parafollicular cells.

3. Occurs in association with MEN type IIA syndrome.

4. TSH suppression is an important part of treatment .

5. Histology characteristically shows 'Orphan Annie' type cells.

PAEDIATRIC DISORDERS

3.51 Oesophageal atresia:
A. Is a congenital abnormality.
B. Is not associated with tracheo-oesophageal fistula.
C. Can cause hydramnios.
D. Is not associated with other intestinal atresias.
E. Is associated with premature birth.

3.52 Oesophageal atresia:
A. Does not cause pneumonitis.
B. Is not associated with abnormal bone development.
C. May present with tracheo-oesophageal fistulae alone without oesophageal atresia.
D. May present as the infant failing to feed.
E. Mortality increases with delayed diagnosis and surgery.

3.53 Considerations for surgery for oesophageal atresia include:
A. Insertion of a feeding gastrostomy.
B. Primary anastomosis of the two oesophageal segments.
C. The operation is always performed in two stages.
D. Closure of tracheo-oesophageal fistulae may not be necessary.
E. Contrast studies are rarely helpful in the planning of surgery.

3.54 The following are true of pyloric stenosis:
A. It may present as a failure to thrive.
B. Vomiting is projectile in nature.
C. The pylorus may be palpable in the left upper quadrant.
D. Peristaltic waves of the small bowel wall may be visible.
E. It is more common in girls.

3.55 The following should be noted in managing pyloric stenosis:
A. Barium meal is the most helpful imaging modality.
B. The pylorus undergoes hyperplasia.
C. There may be a genetic disorder.
D. Ultrasound scan may aid diagnosis.
E. Infants are usually dehydrated and malnourished.

3.56 In pyloric stenosis:
A. Metabolic acidosis is a common biochemical abnormality.
B. Surgery must be carried out immediately upon diagnosis without further fluid resuscitation.
C. Surgery involves the splitting of the entire muscle coat without breaching the mucosa.
D. Duodenal perforation is a complication of Ramstedt's procedure.

3.57 The following are also true of pyloric stenosis:
A. Balloon dilatation has largely replaced pyloromyotomy as the first line treatment.
B. The condition rarely recurs after surgery.
C. Feeding should only be started 24 h after pyloromyotomy.
D. The pyloromyotomy must not include the gastric wall.

3.58 The following statements concerning Hirschsprung's disease are true:
A. The anal canal is always involved.
B. The myenteric plexus ganglion cells are missing.
C. The diseased segment commonly involves the sigmoid colon.
D. It is a common cause of intestinal obstruction in 5–10-year-olds.

3.59 In the management of Hirschsprung's disease, note the following:
A. It is more common in males.
B. Barium enema examination is not possible.
C. Rectal biopsy is rarely helpful.
D. It should not be treated initially with colostomy alone.
E. The definitive operation is excision of the diseased segment with primary anastomosis.

3.60 The following statements are true of meconium ileus:
- A. It is associated with cystic fibrosis.
- B. It is an example of mechanical obstruction.
- C. The meconium is typically impacted in the duodenum.
- D. Gastrograffin enema shows a collapsed colon.
- E. Treatment is by surgical removal of the meconium plug.

3.61 In cases of neonatal volvulus:
- A. There is an association with congenital malrotation of the bowel.
- B. The caecum is rarely involved.
- C. The sigmoid is commonly involved.
- D. Ladd's bands, which are associated with the volvulus segment, can cause duodenal obstruction.
- E. Surgery is always required.

3.62 In cases of imperforate anus:
- A. The defect may be in any part of the colon and rectum.
- B. Rectal defects occur more commonly than anal defects in both sexes.
- C. Rectovaginal or rectourethral fistulae may be present.
- D. The levator ani group of muscles is an important landmark.
- E. Anal defects do not usually require sphincter reconstruction.

3.63 Exomphalos:
- A. Is usually covered by an intact membrane.
- B. Is an example of congenital hernia.
- C. Is not associated with malrotation of the bowel .
- D. Is associated with abnormalities of other organs such as the heart.
- E. Should not be treated surgically if the defect is small.

3.64 The following statements concerning gastroschisis are correct:
- A. The abdominal contents are spilled out of the cavity via a defect in the abdominal wall.
- B. It is usually covered by an intact membrane.
- C. It is more commonly associated with abnormalities of other organs such as the heart than exomphalos.
- D. The defect is usually small.
- E. Surgical repair is always necessary.

3.65 The following are true of umbilical hernias:
A. The umbilical defect usually closes within the first week of life.
B. It is less common in premature babies.
C. Most hernias do not close spontaneously.
D. Any surgery should be delayed until the age of three.
E. Rarely causes intestinal obstruction.

3.66 Concerning intussusception:
A. It is the most common cause of abdominal pain in the neonate.
B. The apex may be a polyp or Meckel's diverticulum.
C. The terminal ileum is most commonly affected.
D. Inflamed Peyer's patches may form the apex.
E. Females are more commonly affected than males.

3.67 In cases of intussusception:
A. Colicky abdominal pain is a common presenting complaint.
B. The affected bowel is not usually palpable.
C. 'Redcurrant jelly' stool may be passed.
D. Vomiting is projectile in nature.
E. The abdomen may be scaphoid.

3.68 In the management of intussusception:
A. Plain X-rays are contraindicated.
B. Barium enema examination is the diagnostic test of choice.
C. Barium enema should not be used as a therapeutic procedure.
D. Hydrostatic reduction should be tried initially.
E. Surgical reduction never involves resection of the affected segment of bowel.

3.69 Meckel's diverticulum:
A. Is present in 4% of the population.
B. Is a remnant of the vitello-intestinal duct.
C. Rarely contains ectopic tissue.
D. May cause abdominal pain when inflamed.
E. Always presents with haemorrhage.

3.70 In the management of Meckel's diverticulum:
A. Peptic ulcers in and around the diverticulum are caused by ectopic pancreatic tissue.
B. Haemorrhage is a common complication of peptic ulcers at this site.
C. Barium meal is the best diagnostic tool.
D. Radioactive technetium can be used to diagnose ectopic gastric mucosa.
E. Those which are incidentally found at laparotomy should always be excised to prevent further complications.

3.71 Wilms' tumour:
A. Is derived from the fetal neural crest cells
B. Usually presents as an abdominal mass in adolescence
C. Rarely needs surgery.
D. Always requires chemo- or radiotherapy for all tumours.
E. Should be staged by selective angiography, which is the most useful tool for this.

3.72 The following are true of torsion of the testicle:
A. It is a surgical emergency.
B. Torsion of the hydatid of Morgagni may cause testicular infarction.
C. It may be caused by epididymo-orchitis.
D. It may present as abdominal pain with nausea and vomiting.
E. The unaffected side should always be fixed to the scrotal wall at surgery.

3.73 Congenital inguinal hernia:
A. Is caused by a patent processus vaginalis.
B. Should be repaired with a mesh.
C. May close without surgical intervention.
D. May be bilateral.
E. Should be repaired within the first year of life.

3.74 In cases of congenital diaphragmatic hernia:
A. Postero-lateral defect is the most common.
B. Patients present with respiratory distress.
C. Scaphoid abdomen and displaced apex beat are common clinical signs.
D. Intubation should be delayed until the patient is on the operating table and ready for surgery.
E. Pulmonary hypoplasia may be present.

3.75 In neonates:
A. The daily water requirements for maintenance is 300 ml/kg.
B. The minimum urine output should be 1 ml/kg/h.
C. The daily amino acid requirement is 2 g/kg.
D. The total daily calorie intake should be about 100 kcal/kg.

3.76 Theme: Neonatal respiratory distress

Options:
A. Pneumonia
B. Diaphragmatic hernia
C. Oesophageal atresia
D. Cystic fibrosis
E. Tetralogy of Fallot
F. Choanal atresia

For each of the patients described below, select the single most likely diagnosis from the list of options above. Each option may be used once, more than once or not at all.

1. A neonate presenting with progressive cyanosis from immediately after birth. The cyanosis seems to be improved and relieved by episodes of crying.

2. A neonate who presents several hours after birth with noisy and rattly breathing, and frothy mucus in the nose and mouth. Hydramnios was present during pregnancy.

3. A neonate presenting with increased respiratory distress and cyanosis. Examination reveals an apex beat displaced to the right and a scaphoid-shaped abdomen.

3.77 Theme: Vomiting in the newborn

Options:
A. Meckel's diverticulum
B. Pyloric stenosis
C. Duodenal atresia
D. Intussusception
E. Diaphragmatic hernia
F. Meconium ileus

For each of the patients described below, select the single most likely diagnosis from the list of options above. Each option may be used once, more than once or not at all.

1. A male child presenting at three weeks of age with projectile vomiting and failure to thrive. He is able to feed and appears hungry after vomiting. Examination reveals a 2 cm long sausage-shaped mass in the epigastrium.

2. A child with Down syndrome presents with vomiting of bile-stained fluid. Erect abdominal X-ray shows a double bubble in the right upper quadrant.

3. A child presents with abdominal distension and bilious vomiting. Another child in the family has cystic fibrosis. Abdominal X-ray shows dilated loops of small bowel.

Abdomen

4.1 Right inguinal hernias:
   A. Commonly strangulate in premature infants.
   B. Are more common in patients who have undergone appendicectomy.
   C. May contain sigmoid colon.
   D. Strangulate more frequently than left inguinal hernias.
   E. Of Littre's type may contain the appendix.

4.2 Ileostomy is associated with:
   A. Depression in at least 10% of patients.
   B. Parastomal fistula as a result of poor surgical technique.
   C. Prolapse, predominantly in loop stomata.
   D. Hypernatraemia because of high output.
   E. A cumulative complication rate of > 50% over ten years.

4.3 Villous atrophy in the small bowel:
   A. May be caused by Chagas' disease.
   B. May improve with a gluten-free diet.
   C. Is usually diagnosed using the Crosbie capsule examination.
   D. Is associated with B-cell lymphoma when caused by coeliac disease.
   C. Is a precursor of intestinal metaplasia.

4.4 In large bowel obstruction:
   A. Small bowel dilatation is seen on abdominal X-ray 50% of the time.
   B. The obstructing lesion is not infrequently found in the rectum.
   C. Vomiting is an early feature.
   D. Electrolyte imbalance is unlikely because the bowel functions normally.
   E. Pseudo-obstruction can be excluded on plain abdominal X-ray.

4.5 Mesenteric venous occlusion:

A. May present insidiously over several days or weeks.

B. Is treated by mesenteric venous thrombectomy.

C. Is associated with the progesterone-only pill.

D. May resolve spontaneously.

E. May be associated with Leiden V deficiency.

4.6 Low anterior resection with total mesorectal excision for rectal cancer at 6 cm from anal verge:

A. Has a higher local recurrence rate than abdomino-perineal resection.

B. Should be performed with the patient in the Lloyd-Thomas position.

C. May cause ejaculatory difficulty.

D. Always requires defunctioning proximal stoma.

E. Should be preceded by chemoradiation for improved survival rates.

4.7 Laparoscopic cholecystectomy:

A. Is safer than open operation for patients with cardiorespiratory disease.

B. Is contraindicated in acute cholecystitis.

C. Is associated with a higher rate of bile duct injury than open cholecystectomy.

D. Is less invasive than open cholecystectomy.

4.8 The stomach:

A. Receives its entire arterial supply from the coeliac trunk.

B. Herniates from the abdominal cavity during development.

C. Is the main source of cholecystokinin.

D. Is related to the left vagus anteriorly and the right vagus posteriorly.

E. Is a common site of gastrointestinal B-cell lymphoma.

4.9 Carcinoma of the oesophagus:

A. Has an overall five-year survival rate of 20%.

B. Is more common in females in the UK.

C. Is rare in patients with tylosis.

D. Responds well to chemotherapy.

E. Is associated with a high salt intake.

4.10 Gastric outlet obstruction:
A. Is a common presentation of peptic ulceration in Western civilizations.
B. Causes metabolic hyperchloraemic alkalosis.
C. May cause Trousseau's sign.
D. May be a complication of ERCP.
E. In children is usually the result of intussusception.

4.11 Acute pancreatitis:
A. Has an overall mortality of 10%.
B. May be related to bendrofluazide.
C. May be caused by seatbelt trauma.
D. Is commonly caused by *E. coli* infection.
E. Plasma amylase level is a good indicator of the severity of inflammation.

4.12 Gastric linitis plastica:
A. Commonly presents with acute GI bleeding.
B. Is characterized by the presence of signet ring cells.
C. Is associated with *Helicobacter pylori* infection.
D. Has a good prognosis.
E. Is frequently misdiagnosed on endoscopy.

4.13 The inguinal canal:
A. Contains the iliohypogastric nerve.
B. Is about 2 cm long in the full-term neonate.
C. Extends from the mid-inguinal point to the pubic tubercle.
D. Contains the round ligament of the ovary.
E. Usually contains the testis in the 39-week male foetus.

4.14 Faecal incontinence in the elderly:
A. Is usually the result of anorectal malignancy.
B. Is contributed to by abnormal anorectal sensory pathways.
C. May be treated by a low residue diet and glycerine suppositories.
D. May be caused by obstetric trauma.
E. Has long-term success when treated by post-anal repair.

4.15 Carcinoid tumours:
A. Are associated with raised urinary VMA.
B. Are characteristically slow growing.
C. May present to respiratory physicians.
D. Cause facial flushing similar in appearance to rosacea.
E. Commonly metastasize to the brain.

4.16 Hepatic colorectal metastases:
A. Mainly present in the right lobe.
B. Commonly cause jaundice.
C. Are inoperable when greater than five in number.
D. May be treated by radiotherapy.
E. Are supplied predominantly by the portal vein.

4.17 Carcinoma of the gallbladder:
A. Is the third most common GI malignancy.
B. Is associated with cholesterol gallstones.
C. Has a good prognosis.
D. Is highly radiosensitive.
E. Is a recognized complication of long-term treatment with NSAIDs.

4.18 Raised alkaline phosphatase may be caused by:
A. Choledocholithiasis.
B. The oral contraceptive pill.
C. A complication of ulcerative colitis.
D. Osteomalacia.
E. Osteoporosis.

4.19 In patients with ulcerative colitis:
A. Colonic cancer will develop at 2% per year after ten years of disease if it involves the whole colon.
B. Toxic megacolon is always an indication for surgery.
C. Extraintestinal manifestations may be an indication for colectomy.
D. Panproctocolectomy should be performed for fulminant total colitis.
E. The disease is worsened by smoking.

4.20 The following statements concerning splenectomy are correct:
  A. With currently available surgical techniques, it is rarely indicated in trauma.
  B. It should not be performed until puberty for haematological disorders.
  C. It predisposes to sepsis predominantly from Gram-negative bacterial cell wall toxins.
  D. It should be preceded by vaccination with pneumovax, *Haemophilus influenzae* and influenza vaccines.
  E. It may be performed laparoscopically for trauma.

4.21 Chylous ascites:
  A. May be diagnosed by visual inspection of fluid obtained from ascitic tap.
  B. Is a recognized complication of cholecystectomy.
  C. May be a presenting feature of pancreatic carcinoma.
  D. May complicate abdominal aortic aneurysm repair.
  E. May be treated with a diet high in protein, carbohydrate and medium-chain triglycerides.

4.22 The oesophagus:
  A. Consists of four layers: mucosa, submucosa, a muscular layer and serosa.
  B. Passes through the diaphragm at T12.
  C. Is crossed by the azygos vein just below the tracheal bifurcation.
  D. Is supplied by a branch of the thyrocervical trunk in the upper third.
  E. Is atretic in 1:2500 live births.

4.23 Gastro-oesophageal reflux disease:
  A. May present with dental erosion.
  B. Is common in Asia.
  C. Commonly causes recurrent pneumonia in adults.
  D. Is graded in severity by McMaster's score.
  E. May be diagnosed with Bernstein's acid perfusion test.

4.24 Achalasia of the oesophagus:
A. Is characterized by failure of relaxation of the lower oesophageal sphincter and absent peristalsis in the oesophageal body.
B. Has been treated with Botulinum toxin injection.
C. After treatment with Heller's cardiomyotomy may result in gastro-oesophageal reflux.
D. Is commoner in males than females.
E. May cause similar radiological appearance to chronic infection with *Trypanosoma cruzi*.

4.25 Massive lower gastrointestinal bleeding:
A. Settles spontaneously in 80–90%.
B. Should be investigated by emergency colonoscopy.
C. Is usually a result of carcinoma in the elderly.
D. Is rarely caused by angiodysplasia.
E. Is not usually helped by angiography if bleeding is less than l ml/min.

4.26 Acute acalculous cholecystitis:
A. Is most commonly seen in middle-aged women with constipation.
B. Is thought to be caused by splanchnic ischaemia.
C. May be treated by percutaneous cholecystostomy.
D. Is usually caused by clostridium infection.
E. Is related to gallbladder cancer.

4.27 Non-surgical treatment of gallstones:
A. Is suitable for radiolucent stones less than 1 cm in diameter.
B. Is usually achieved with a three-month course of ursodeoxycholic acid for cholesterol stones.
C. May be undertaken with MTBE.
D. Is recommended for young patients awaiting renal transplant.
E. Has a low incidence of recurrent stones after medical dissolution.

4.28 Cholangiocarcinoma:
   A. Represents approximately 1% of all gastrointestinal cancer.
   B. Is related to clonorchis sinensis infection.
   C. Is rarely associated with choledocholithiasis.
   D. Metastasizes early.
   E. Presents with obstructive jaundice in 90% of cases.

4.29 Sclerosing cholangitis:
   A. Is associated with Crohn's disease and ulcerative colitis.
   B. Is commoner in females.
   C. May present with fulminant hepatic failure.
   D. Is usually confined to the distal bile duct.
   E. Is associated with cholangiocarcinoma.

4.30 Emergency surgery in the jaundiced patient:
   A. Usually requires replacement of clotting Factor VIII.
   B. Is commonly required for choledocholithiasis.
   C. May result in renal failure because of endotoxaemia.
   D. Is frequently complicated by anaerobic infection.
   E. May be associated with coagulopathy, which can be corrected by preoperative intramuscular Vitamin K.

4.31 The following are true of adenocarcinoma of the pancreas:
   A. Eighty-five per cent of tumours are unresectable at the time of diagnosis.
   B. It has an overall five-year survival of 10%.
   C. It is related to oral contraceptive usage.
   D. CA 19-9 is a highly specific tumour marker.
   E. It may present with peripheral neuropathy.

4.32 Gastrinoma:
   A. Causes peptic ulceration in the distal duodenum and jejunum.
   B. Is rarely malignant.
   C. Is usually easily seen on CT scan of the pancreas.
   D. May be associated with homonymous hemianopia in MEN type II.
   E. May arise in the duodenal wall.

4.33 The following statements concerning portal hypertension and oesophageal varices are correct:
A. In Western societies, they are usually caused by alcohol.
B. They result in caudal lobe hypertrophy in Budd–Chiari syndrome.
C. They should be treated electively by transhepatic portosystemic shunting provided no complications have developed.
D. They result in early mortality from acute variceal haemorrhage in about 50%.
E. If requiring oesophageal transection as an emergency will require reanastomosis within one week.

4.34 Microscopic haematuria:
A. In a middle-aged male with lower abdominal pain is likely to be the result of urinary tract infection.
B. May occur in patients with acute diverticulitis.
C. May be related to exercise.
D. In a catheter specimen of urine is suggestive of urinary tract pathology.
E. Is frequently asymptomatic.

4.35 Raised plasma amylase:
A. May be asymptomatic.
B. May occur in a ruptured ectopic pregnancy.
C. May occur in renal impairment.
D. That is greater than five times normal can only be caused by acute pancreatitis.
E. In combination with gas in the portal vein suggests intestinal ischaemia.

4.36 Regarding perianal sepsis:
A. Recurrence of a previously drained abscess is highly suggestive of Crohn's disease.
B. Culture of pus is helpful in predicting the presence of a fistula.
C. A high fistula identified at the time of abscess drainage should be laid open.
D. Extrasphincteric fistulae should be treated with a seton.
E. A loose seton is used to mark a high fistula tract and allow drainage of pus prior to definitive treatment.

4.37 Haemorrhoids:
A. Are varicose veins of the anal canal.
B. May be treated by sphincterotomy.
C. May be injected with phenol in oil to produce fibrosis.
D. When thrombosed should be treated by incision and drainage.
E. May be treated by haemorrhoidectomy but weeping from the anus can continue for six weeks in the normal postoperative course.

4.38 Adaptation of the bowel to massive small bowel resection:
A. May occur in the early postoperative period while the patient is parenterally fed.
B. Is better after jejunal than ileal resection.
C. Is inhibited by steroids.
D. Is stimulated by monosaccharides to a greater extent than dissaccharides.
E. Is more likely to occur if the ileocaecal valve is preserved.

4.39 Femoral hernia:
A. Is five times as common in women as men.
B. Emerges below and lateral to the pubic tubercle.
C. Not infrequently resembles a metastatic inguinal node from rectal cancer.
D. According to Royal College guidelines should be repaired with mesh.
E. May be differentiated from a saphena varix by the presence of a cough impulse.

4.40 Umbilical hernia in children:
A. Is commoner in infants with Down syndrome.
B. Strangulates in 2% of cases.
C. Commonly closes spontaneously up to five years of age.
D. Requires surgical repair if greater than 2 cm in diameter at the age of one year.
E. Should be repaired with mesh if greater than 2 cm.

4.41 Differential diagnoses of an inguinal hernia include:
   A. Femoral hernia.
   B. Vaginal hydrocele.
   C. Undescended testis.
   D. Ectopic testis.
   E. Psoas abscess.

4.42 Inguinal hernias in children:
   A. Are commoner in premature and low birthweight babies.
   B. Occur in both sexes.
   C. Are commoner in males.
   D. Are present at birth but may present later.
   E. Are caused by increased intra-abdominal pressure.

4.43 Femoral hernias:
   A. In females are as common as inguinal hernias.
   B. Are lateral to the femoral vein.
   C. Have a higher risk of strangulation.
   D. Are repaired operatively by the Lichtenstein method.
   E. May give no previous history of a hernia in patients with strangulation.

4.44 Operative techniques for repair of inguinal hernias include:
   A. Herniotomy only.
   B. Bassini repair.
   C. Shouldice repair.
   D. Lichtenstein repair.
   E. Stoppa repair.
   F. Laparoscopic repair.

4.45 With regards to inguinal hernias:
   A. Mortality of elective repair is 5–10 times lower than emergency repair of strangulated hernias.
   B. Richter's hernia is a partial enterocoele and results in strangulation and obstruction.
   C. Surgical repair necessitates overnight stay in hospital if done under general anaesthetic.
   D. Use of absorbable mesh is advised in surgical repair.
   E. Following repair patients are advised to avoid sports for a year.

4.46 The femoral canal:
A. Lies medial to the femoral vein.
B. Has the inguinal ligament as its anterior border.
C. Has the lacunar ligament as its lateral border.
D. Has the pectineal ligament as its posterior border.
E. Contains the lymph node of Cloquet.

4.47 Regarding the repair of abdominal wall hernias:
A. Almost 100 000 hernia operations are performed annually in the UK.
B. The hernial contents form part of the sac wall in a sliding hernia.
C. The cremasteric muscle forms part of the posterior wall repair.
D. Persistent groin pain may be due to ilioinguinal nerve entrapment.
E. Injury to the genito-femoral nerve results in weakness of the dartos muscle.

4.48 A strangulated inguinal hernia causing intestinal obstruction:
A. Is best treated by attempted manual reduction.
B. Is a surgical emergency requiring prompt surgical intervention.
C. Is an indication for laparotomy.
D. Cannot be repaired by mesh insertion.
E. Is managed during the first 48 h with intravenous fluids and nasogastric tube.

4.49 Causes of non-specific acute abdominal pain include:
A. Irritable bowel syndrome.
B. Viral infections.
C. Gastroenteritis.
D. Nerve root pain.
E. Psychosomatic pain.

4.50 Regarding blood tests and acute abdominal pain:
  A. With the exception of serum amylase, other tests have doubtful diagnostic significance.
  B. A single measurement of white blood count is as useful as serial measurement.
  C. Estimation of acid–base status is helpful in the diagnosis of intestinal ischaemia.
  D. High C reactive protein levels are diagnostic of peritonitis.
  E. Normal liver function tests excludes the presence of gallstones.

4.51 In the management of acute abdominal pain:
  A. An erect plain chest X-ray is the most appropriate investigation for detection of free intraperitoneal gas.
  B. An erect abdominal X-ray is necessary to diagnose intestinal obstruction.
  C. No detectable gas under the diaphragm on the erect CXR excludes perforated viscus.
  D. Abdominal ultrasound examination is most appropriate to exclude pancreatitis.
  E. Urgent urine microscopy is unnecessary.

4.52 Signs of successful resuscitation of hypovolaemic shock caused by intestinal obstruction include:
  A. Improved level of consciousness.
  B. Slowing of tachycardia.
  C. Decreasing abdominal girth.
  D. Decreasing NG aspirate.
  E. Improved capillary return.

4.53 In acute gastrointestinal diseases:
  A. Diarrhoea and loss of colonic mucus may cause hyperkalaemia.
  B. Gastrointestinal fluid losses are best replaced with crystalloids.
  C. Low serum sodium must be corrected before surgical intervention.
  D. A healthy adult may lose up to 1500 ml of fluid before physical signs are obvious.
  E. Inadequately treated fluid loss is a common cause of multiple organ failure.

4.54 Peutz–Jeghers syndrome:
    A. Is an autosomal recessive condition.
    B. Often presents with anaemia in childhood.
    C. Is characterized by circumoral mucocutaneous pigmented lesions.
    D. Is associated with adenomatous polyps of the small intestine.
    E. Malignant change occurs in 2–3% of polyps.

4.55 About peptic ulceration:
    A. *Helicobacter pylori* is a Gram-positive bacillus.
    B. Duodenal is more common than oesophageal ulceration.
    C. Zollinger–Ellison syndrome is associated with gastric hyposecretion.
    D. Proton pump inhibitors (PPIs) will heal 95% of duodenal ulcers in six weeks.
    E. Triple therapy (omeprazole, metronidazole and ampicillin) can eradicate *H. pylori*.

4.56 Pancreatic carcinomas:
    A. Present with pain, weight loss and obstructive jaundice.
    B. Occur in the head of the gland in less than 20% of cases.
    C. Are ductal adenocarcinomas in 90% of cases.
    D. Are solely detected by ultrasound.
    E. Are mostly unsuitable for curative surgery.

4.57 The following statements are true of acute appendicitis:
    A. It is commonest in childhood.
    B. Mortality increases with age and is greatest in the elderly.
    C. The commonest lie of the appendix is in a retrocaecal position.
    D. Faecoliths may be present in resected specimens.
    E. Appendicitis is a possible diagnosis in the absence of pyrexia.

4.58 Gallbladder stones:
- A. Are mostly composed of cholesterol.
- B. As pigment stones are caused by increased excretion of polymerized conjugated bilirubin.
- C. Are not a risk factor for the development of gallbladder carcinoma.
- D. Are radio-opaque.
- E. Impacted in Hartmann's pouch cause mucocele of the gallbladder.

4.59 Common bile duct calculi:
- A. Are found in over 10% of patients undergoing cholecystectomy.
- B. Can present with Charcot's triad.
- C. Are suggested by a bile duct diameter > 8 mm on ultrasound.
- D. Are best treated by ERCP, sphincterotomy and balloon clearance.
- E. If removed by open exploration of the common bile duct, the T-tube can safely be removed after three days.

4.60 Ulcerative colitis:
- A. Affects the full thickness of the colon wall.
- B. Always involves the rectum.
- C. May affect the terminal ileal (backwash ileitis).
- D. Commonly causes enterocutaneous fistulae.
- E. Spares the serosa of the colon.

4.61 Regarding surgery for ulcerative colitis:
- A. Patients with total colitis will require surgery within four years to prevent malignant transformation.
- B. Panproctocolectomy and pouch formation is appropriate as an emergency operation.
- C. Pouches can be fashioned as 'S', 'J' or 'W' loops.
- D. Patients with a successful pouch are continent for stools.
- E. With a pouch the mean stool frequency is about ten times per day.

4.62 Anal fissures:
- **A.** Commonly occur in the posterior midline of the rectum.
- **B.** Suggest Crohn's disease if they recur.
- **C.** May heal with the use of a bulking agent.
- **D.** Treated by sphincterotomy could lead to incontinence.
- **E.** Should be treated by sphincterotomy as this is safer than Lord's procedure.

4.63 Familial adenomatous polyposis:
- **A.** Is inherited as an autosomal recessive condition.
- **B.** Is characterized by polyp formation in late adulthood.
- **C.** Is associated with osteomas and epidermoid cysts in Gardner syndrome.
- **D.** Is caused by a mutation on the short arm of chromosome 12.
- **E.** Can be screened for by rigid or flexible sigmoidoscopy.

4.64 The following are true of rectal cancer:
- **A.** It is predisposed by metaplastic polyps.
- **B.** Local recurrence is unaffected by total mesorectal excision.
- **C.** In the upper third of the rectum is most appropriately managed by an abdomino-perineal resection.
- **D.** The rectum is the commonest site of colorectal tumours.
- **E.** Chemotherapy is of proven benefit in Dukes' A tumours.

4.65 Oesophageal cancer:
- **A.** Can be eradicated by large-scale screening programmes.
- **B.** Arises most commonly in Barrett's oesophagus.
- **C.** Incidence is related to environmental factors.
- **D.** Is not curable surgically.
- **E.** Palliation with a metallic stent is rarely successful.

4.66 Indications for surgery in acute duodenal ulcer haemorrhage include:
A. Failure of endoscopic control of active bleeding.
B. Recurrent bleeding after endoscopic control.
C. Age over 60 and transfusion of more than four units of blood.
D. Large ulcer in the posterior wall.

4.67 Emergency surgery for bleeding duodenal ulcer entails:
A. Truncal vagotomy and pyloroplasty after control of bleeding.
B. Cauterization of the bleeding vessel.
C. Partial gastrectomy and selective vagotomy.
D. Underunning of the bleeding vessel with no vagotomy.
E. Pylorus-preserving duodenectomy.

4.68 Causes of acute life-threatening colonic bleeding include:
A. Hamartomas.
B. Angiodysplasia.
C. Diverticulosis.
D. Ischaemic colitis.
E. Ulcerative colitis.

4.69 Colonic angiodysplasia:
A. May be an incidental finding in approximately 3–6% of all colonoscopies.
B. Is associated with cardiac valvular disease.
C. Only presents with acute gastrointestinal bleeding.
D. Affects the right colon only in 60–80% of cases.
E. Is only diagnosed by angiography.

4.70 Causes of small bowel obstruction include:
A. Crohn's disease.
B. Previous abdominal surgery.
C. Diaphragmatic hernias.
D. Carcinoma of the caecum.
E. Carcinoma of the rectum.

4.71 Small bowel obstruction typically presents with:
 A. Central colicky abdominal pain.
 B. Pyrexia.
 C. Signs of localized peritonitis.
 D. Abdominal distension and vomiting.
 E. Inaudible bowel sounds.

4.72 Management of small bowel obstruction includes:
 A. Urinary catherization.
 B. No analgesia as it may mask impending peritonitis.
 C. Rectal enemas.
 D. Slow fluid resuscitation to prevent heart failure.
 E. Replacement of nasogastric tube fluid loss.

4.73 In small bowel obstruction as a result of groin hernias:
 A. Gangrene and small bowel resection are very rare.
 B. Surgery is mandatory.
 C. A midline laparotomy is always necessary.
 D. A direct surgical approach to the hernia is appropriate.
 E. Marlex mesh is contraindicated to repair the hernia.

4.74 Acute appendicitis:
 A. Is the commonest intra-abdominal surgical emergency.
 B. Has a peak incidence in the 45–55 age group.
 C. Is caused by bacterial invasion of the appendicular mucosa.
 D. That results in an appendicular mass is best managed conservatively in an unstable ill patient.
 E. Is accurately diagnosed by ultrasound scanning.

4.75 Perforated peptic ulcer:
 A. Incidence is rising
 B. Can be the result of steroid therapy.
 C. Can be managed conservatively in fit patients who show a persistent leak on gastrograffin meal.
 D. Can be treated laparoscopically.
 E. Presents with pnuemoperitonium in over 90% of cases.

4.76 The following statements are true when investigating massive rectal bleeding (non-haemorrhoidal) of unknown site in an unstable patient:
A. Gastroscopy should be performed first.
B. Colonoscopy should be performed first.
C. Immediate laparotomy is mandatory.
D. Mesenteric angiography should be done first.
E. Labelled red-cell scan is useful.

4.77 Presenting features of sepsis and systemic inflammatory response syndrome (SIRS) include:
A. Haemorrhage and bruising.
B. Lactic acidosis.
C. Acute respiratory distress syndrome.
D. Hyperthermia.
E. Hypothermia.

4.78 Multiple organ dysfunction syndrome (MODS) can be defined by several parameters which include:
A. Mean arterial pressure less than 49 mmHg.
B. WBC more than 20 000 mm^3.
C. Dependence on mechanical ventilation for more than 12 h.
D. Oliguria less than 5 ml/kg/h.
E. Glasgow Coma Scale score less than 8.

4.79 Factors contributing to the development of MODS include:
A. Uncontrolled sepsis.
B. Massive resuscitation.
C. Hypovolaemic shock.
D. Specific organ disease.
E. Crush injuries.

4.80 The following statements are true:
A. Some patients are more susceptible to septic complications than others.
B. Systemic inflammatory response syndrome (SIRS) is thought to be a result of inadequate or overwhelmed local host defence mechanisms.
C. SIRS responds to intravenous antibiotic therapy.
D. SIRS results from infection only.
E. When bacterial in origin, sepsis and SIRS are synonymous.

4.81 Theme: Altered bowel habit and rectal bleeding

Options :
A. Diverticulitis
B. Rectal carcinoma
C. Colonic adenomata/polyps
D. Crohn's disease
E. Ulcerative colitis

For each of the patients described below, select the single most likely diagnosis from the list of options above. Each option may be used once, more than once or not at all.

1. A 70-year-old male patient presents with diarrhoea and fresh rectal bleeding for one month. He experiences occasional abdominal pain and loss of appetite.

2. A 28-year-old female comes into Outpatients' with central abdominal pains, bloodstained diarrhoea and anaemia. She has no relevant past medical history.

4.82 Theme: Antibiotic prophylaxis

Options:
A. Augmentin
B. Piperacillin
C. Teicoplanin
D. Cefuroxime and metronidazole
E. Cotrimoxazole
F. Ciprofloxacin
G. Clindamycin
H. None of the above

From the options above choose the most appropriate antibiotic prophylaxis for the following surgical patients. Each answer may be used once, more than once or not at all.

1. A 65-year-old male patient undergoing PTFE femoro-distal bypass graft.

2. An 80-year-old man about to undergo prostatic biopsy.

3. A 63-year-old woman prepared for sigmoid colectomy.

4.83 Theme: Sutures

Options:
A. No. 1 loop nylon
B. 4/0 vicryl
C. 2/0 PDS
D. 2/0 prolene
E. 6/0 ethilon
F. 4/0 Goretex
G. 3/0 chromic catgut

For each of the anastomoses below choose the most appropriate suture from those listed above. Each answer may be used once, more than once or not at all.

1. Adominal aorta to Dacron graft.

2. Gastrojejunostomy.

Urinary system and renal transplantation

URINARY SYSTEM

5.1 Transitional cell carcinoma of the bladder:
   A. Is best diagnosed by computed tomography (CT).
   B. Commonly causes microscopic or macroscopic haematuria.
   C. Has a higher incidence in smokers.
   D. Commonly metastasizes in a retrograde fashion via the ureters to involve the renal parenchyma.
   E. Carries a worse prognosis in the presence of coexisting carcinoma in situ of the bladder.

5.2 Patients presenting with macroscopic haematuria should:
   A. Receive bladder irrigation via a three-way urethral catheter.
   B. Have their urine sent for microscopy, culture and sensitivity.
   C. Undergo cystoscopy.
   D. Have a radionuclide renogram.
   E. Have an intravenous urogram (IVU) and/or ultrasound of the renal tract.

5.3 The ureter is:
   A. Widest at the vesico-ureteric junction.
   B. Lined by transitional cell epithelium.
   C. The commonest site involved in transitional cell carcinoma of the urinary tract.
   D. Anterior to the uterine artery.
   E. Totally dependent on the autonomic nervous system for its peristaltic activity.

5.4 **An unwell patient with an 8 mm upper ureteric stone causing ureteric obstruction and a pyrexia of c. 39.5°C should:**
   A. Receive urgent extracorporeal lithotripsy (ESWL) to fragment the stone and relieve the obstruction.
   B. Have urine sent for microscopy, culture and sensitivity.
   C. Have a urethral catheter inserted to exclude bladder outflow obstruction.
   D. Have blood culture taken.
   E. Undergo emergency ureteroscopy and lithoclast treatment to the stone under antibiotic cover.

5.5 **Bladder calculi are:**
   A. Best treated surgically with concomitant treatment of bladder outflow obstruction.
   B. Usually caused by hyperoxaluria.
   C. Best treated with regular intravesical instillations of Suby's G solution.
   D. Always visualized on a plain KUB (kidney ureter bladder) X-ray.
   E. Usually composed of uric acid or struvite (magnesium, ammonium and phosphate triple stone).

5.6 **Urinary frequency and urgency:**
   A. Can be caused by bladder outflow obstruction.
   B. May be present in patients suffering from diabetes mellitus.
   C. Should be managed initially by administering an anticholinergic.
   D. Can be triggered by excessive intake of caffeine.
   E. Should always be treated by transurethral resection of the prostate.

5.7 **An enlarged (150 g) benign prostate gland:**
   A. Will always cause more severe symptoms than a 50 g benign prostate.
   B. Is better removed via an open prostatectomy than via transurethral resection.
   C. Is an absolute contraindication to urethral catheterization.
   D. Is a predisposing factor to the subsequent development of adenocarcinoma of the prostate.
   E. Should be treated by an LHRH (luteinizing hormone releasing hormone) analogue before contemplating surgery.

5.8 **Metastatic adenocarcinoma of the prostate:**
   A. Involving the axial skeleton should be treated aggressively by radical prostatectomy followed by antiandrogen therapy and radiotherapy to the bony metastases.
   B. Is rare in men under 40 years of age.
   C. Causing spinal cord compression should be referred urgently to the palliative care team.
   D. Requires high-dose stilboestrol as first-line treatment in a symptomatic patient.
   E. When treated by bilateral orchidectomy requires initial antiandrogen therapy to prevent 'tumour flare'.

5.9 **Prostate specific antigen (PSA):**
   A. In the serum rises significantly after digital rectal examination.
   B. Is specific to the prostate gland and absent from other tissues of the body.
   C. Is always elevated in adenocarcinoma of the prostate.
   D. Is a hormone involved in the regulation of the growth of the prostate.
   E. Is a serine protease involved in the liquefaction of semen.

5.10 Benign prostatic hyperplasia (BPH):
A. Always involves the whole of the prostate gland.
B. Involves only the glandular but not the stromal element of the gland.
C. Commonly involves the external urethral sphincter and causes bladder outflow obstruction.
D. Can cause a rise in prostate specific antigen (PSA).
E. Usually begins in adolescence.

5.11 Regarding testicular torsion:
A. Extravaginal torsion usually occurs in adults.
B. Intravaginal torsion is most commonly seen in adolescents.
C. Elevation of a torted testicle will usually relieve the pain.
D. The testicle usually twists medially.
E. Leydig cell function is more resistant to hypoxia than spermatogenesis.

5.12 The following can cause acute urinary retention in men:
A. Spinal cord compression.
B. Acute prostatitis.
C. Urethral stricture.
D. Beta-blockers.
E. Epidural anaesthesia.

5.13 Bladder outflow obstruction in men:
A. Is always associated with a large post-void residual.
B. Is likely to be present in a man with a flow rate < 10 ml/s.
C. Can be caused by sphincter dyssynergia.
D. Can be easily diagnosed from lower urinary tract symptoms.
E. Can be caused by ureteric strictures.

5.14 In blunt renal trauma:
  A. Microscopic haematuria in a cardiovascularly and neurologically stable patient requires no further imaging.
  B. Frank haematuria should be investigated with an intravenous urogram or contrast CT once the patient has been resuscitated.
  C. Most injuries are contusions or minor parenchymal tears that can be treated conservatively.
  D. Injuries associated with large haematomas should usually be explored by laparotomy.
  E. The absence of blood in the urine excludes any renal injury.

5.15 The following are associated with vesico-ureteric reflux:
  A. Infection.
  B. Complete duplication of the collecting systems.
  C. Medial placement of ureteric orifices.
  D. Old age.
  E. Short submucosal ureteric tunnel.

5.16 Theme: Disorders of prostate

Options:
A. Bladder-neck stenosis
B. Spinal cord compression secondary to metastasis from adenocarcinoma of the prostate
C. Obstructive uropathy
D. Chronic prostatitis
E. Prostatodynia
F. Benign prostatic hyperplasia

For each of the patients described below, select the single most likely diagnosis from the list of options above. Each option may be used once, more than once or not at all.

1. A 78-year-old man with recurrence of lower urinary tract symptoms of hesistancy, variable stream and terminal dribbling. He had a transurethral resection of the prostate three years ago during which 9 g of benign tissue was resected. A benign and small prostatic remnant was found on rectal examination and he has a poor flow rate.

2. A 79-year-old man with back pain, lethargy and lower limb weakness. An irregular prostate was noted on rectal examination. There is moderate bilateral lower limb weakness, and a markedly raised prostate specific antigen ($\times$ 100). He has an osteosclerotic lesion in lumbar vertebrae 1 and 2.

3. An 80-year-old man presenting with malaise and drowsiness. He is uraemic with a raised creatinine. He has a palpable bladder and a moderately enlarged prostate on examination. Hb was 9.8 g/dl. Ultrasound revealed bilateral upper tract dilatation with thinning of the renal cortex.

5.17 Theme: Urological disorders

Options:
A. Ureteric calculus
B. Transitional carcinoma of the ureter
C. Transitional carcinoma of the bladder
D. Renal angiolyomyoma
E. Renal cell carcinoma
F. Retroperitoneal fibrosis

For each of the patients described below, select the single most likely diagnosis from the list of options above. Each option may be used once, more than once or not at all.

1. A 54-year-old female presented with frank haematuria and left loin pain. Plain KUB X-ray did not reveal any opacity. Contrast films showed a dilated left pelvicalyceal system and a distended ureter to the level of the vesico-ureteric junction where an irregular filling defect was seen in the bladder.

2. A 23-year-old female presented with frank haematuria and left loin pain. She was hypotensive on arrival but responded to resuscitation with Ringer's lactate solution and remained stable. She has adenoma sebaceum on her face and left loin tenderness on examination. Computer tomography revealed bilateral renal masses composed predominantly of fat.

3. A 60-year-old man was seen in clinic with fever, fatigue, weight loss and bilateral lower limb swelling. Abdominal examination was unremarkable. Slightly irregular outline of upper pole of right kidney on intravenous urogram. Ultrasound revealed a heterogeneous mass in the same region and a large filling defect was seen in the inferior vena cava on computer tomography.

4. A 60-year-old woman presented to the clinic with renal impairment. Ultrasound showed normal renal cortical thickness but dilated pelvicalyceal system bilaterally. In addition, there was medial deviation of the ureters on intravenous urogram. Her ESR was raised.

5. A 70-year-old man developed frank haematuria and clot retention. Examination confirmed a distended bladder and a benign prostate. Intravenous urogram revealed normal upper tract but a large filling defect in the bladder.

5.18 Theme: Transurethral resections

Options:
A. Hypovolaemia secondary to excessive blood loss
B. Transurethral resection (TUR) syndrome
C. Pulmonary embolism
D. Bladder perforation
E. Colovesical fistula

For each of the patients described below, select the single most likely diagnosis from the list of options above. Each option may be used once, more than once or not at all.

1. A 75-year-old man underwent a prolonged transurethral resection of the prostate. He became hypertensive, bradycardiac and confused in the recovery room. His P_aO_2 was 11 kPa on 4 l oxygen/min, Hb 9.8 g/dl, WBC normal, Na 120 mmol/l, K 2.8 mmol/l.

2. A 65-year-old woman underwent a transurethral resection of tumour at the vault of the urinary bladder. She complained of abdominal pain 3 h later. Her lower abdomen was distended and tender but there was no palpable bladder.

5.19 Theme: Scrotum and testicles (I)

Options:
A. Epididymitis
B. Torsion of the testicle
C. Hydrocele
D. Torted appendix testi
E. Inguinal hernia
F. Epididymal cyst

For each of the scenarios described below, select the single most likely answer from the list of options. Each option may be used once, more than once or not at all.

1. A 16-year-old boy with a 4 h history of left testicular pain. On examination the testicle was tender on its superior aspect and a black spot could be visualized through the scrotal skin.

2. A 22-year-old man presenting with a non-painful scrotal swelling. On examination he has a swelling on the left side of the scrotum. The testicle is palpable separately from the swelling, but the swelling does not transilluminate. You cannot get above the swelling.

5.20 Theme: Scrotum and testicles (II)

Options:
A. Seminoma of the testicle
B. Leydig cell tumour
C. Sertoli cell tumour
D. Teratoma of testicle
E. Mixed seminoma/teratoma
F. Hydrocele
G. Sperm granuloma
H. Testicular torsion
I. Ureteric stone
J. Epididymitis

For each of the scenarios described below, select the single most likely answer from the list of options. Each option may be used once more than once or not at all.

1. A 27-year-old man presents with a two-week history of a testicular mass. Ultrasound confirms a homogeneous mass within the body of the testicle. Both the alpha fetoprotein and BHCG are markedly raised.

2. A 30-year-old man with a previous history of undescended testicle presents with a testicular mass. BHCG is raised and the alpha fetoprotein is in the normal range.

3. A 24-year-old man with 3 h history of severe pain, in the left testicle and groin. On examination the testicle is non-tender. Investigations show microscopic haematuria, but no leucocytes or nitrates in the urine.

RENAL TRANSPLANTATION

5.21 Renal transplantation is absolutely contraindicated in:
  A. Oxalosis.
  B. Focal segmental glomerulosclerosis.
  C. Hepatitis C.
  D. HIV positivity.
  E. Chronic pyelonephritis.

5.22 A 40-year old man has chronic renal failure and complains of mild tiredness. The only abnormalities are a slowly rising serum creatinine and blood urea. The following operative procedures are appropriate for preparing this patient for dialysis and future cadaveric renal transplantation:
  A. Insertion of a peritoneal dialysis catheter.
  B. Bilateral nephrectomy.
  C. Surgical creation of an arteriovenous fistula in the forearm.
  D. Cystoscopy.
  E. Renal biopsy.

5.23 With respect to kidney donation by living relatives, the following statements are true:
  A. An adult relative should be chosen because the physiological consequences of nephrectomy are diminished in the adult.
  B. Children should be considered preferentially because the physiologically younger organ has a better chance in normal function.
  C. Siblings should be considered preferentially for immunological reasons.
  D. None of the above.

5.24 The following make a cadaver kidney totally unsuitable for a particular recipient:
  A. ABO incompatibility.
  B. Presence of a current positive T-cell crossmatch.
  C. A historically positive T-cell crossmatch but a current T-cell negative crossmatch.
  D. 60 h of cold ischaemia.
  E. Multiple arteries.

5.25 The following are some of the criteria essential to make a diagnosis of brain death:

A. Absence of significant hypothermia.

B. Apnoea in response to acidosis or hypercarbia.

C. A flat electroencephalogram (EEG).

D. Absence of drug overdosage.

E. Absent corneal or pupillary reflexes.

5.26 A patient receives a cadaver renal transplant without intraoperative incident. While there is good initial function, the urine output drops suddenly following 6 h of good urine output despite a patent urinary catheter. The following statements are true:

A. An attempt at inducing diuresis with large doses of loop diuretics should be made.

B. Surgical exploration should be performed because oliguria in this situation is almost always caused by an arterial or venous thrombosis.

C. Antirejection treatment should be instituted because oliguria indicates hyperacute rejection.

D. Broad-spectrum antibiotics should be started because infection is the most likely cause.

E. None of the above.

5.27 The surgical procedure of renal transplantation requires one or more of the following:

A. Anastomosis – usually to the external iliac or common iliac veins and arteries.

B. Pretransplant assessment of the iliac blood vessels for patency and blood flow through the arteries.

C. Anastomosis to the internal hypogastric artery.

D. Anastomosis of the ureter to the bladder with a non-refluxing technique.

E. Bilateral nephrectomy.

5.28 The following are true concerning immunosuppression in the immune system in renal transplantation:
   A. Viral infections remain the most serious post-transplant problem.
   B. Women should not have children because of the teratogenic effects of immunosuppression.
   C. Patients should not return to work because of their susceptibility to infection.
   D. There is an increased potential for malignancy associated with other oncogenic factors.
   E. None of the above.

5.29 Patients who become pregnant following a successful renal transplant should:
   A. Stop immunosuppression.
   B. Request a termination of the pregnancy.
   C. Monitor progress of the pregnancy carefully and assess renal parameters regularly.
   D. Take extra immunosuppression.
   E. None of the above.

5.30 A renal transplant recipient with good kidney function has an increasing blood pressure. Examination reveals a bruit over the kidney and angiography reveals 80% renal artery stenosis. He should:
   A. Control BP with antihypertensive agents only.
   B. Change immunosuppression.
   C. Receive urgent antirejection treatment.
   D. Have percutaneous balloon angioplasty.
   E. Undergo urgent surgical exploration and correction of the stenosis.

5.31 The following statements are true concerning anti-HLA antibodies:

A. They are associated with hyperacute allograft rejection when directed against donor antigens.

B. They are present when panel cells are not reactive (PRA = 0%)

C. There are multiple specificities present when all panel cells are highly reactive, that is, PRA > 70%.

D. They are most often the result of sensitization to allogenic cells from blood transfusion and previous transplantation.

E. Plasmaphoresis will remove all antibodies from any known recipient

5.32 Which of the following has the greatest long-term patency for use in vascular access for haemodialysis:

A. A surgically created arteriovenous fistula.

B. Saphenous vein placed as a loop in the upper thigh.

C. A percutaneously placed subclavian catheter.

D. A surgically placed internal jugular catheter.

E. A Scribner arteriovenous shunt.

5.33 Absolute contraindications for cadaveric organ donation include:

A. Advanced malignancy.

B. Bacterial sepsis.

C. Severe hypertension.

D. Intravenous drug abuse.

E. HBsAg +ve.

5.34 A 40-year-old patient receiving intermittent peritoneal dialysis presents with severe abdominal pain and a cloudy exchange solution. The following are possible options at various stages in the management of PD peritonitis:

A. Broad-spectrum antibiotic therapy.

B. Laparotomy with removal of the dialysis catheter.

C. Addition of antibiotics to the peritoneal fluid bags and continuing peritoneal dialysis.

D. Conversion to haemodialysis.

5.35 A patient receives a well-matched cadaver donor renal transplant with good initial function. He returns 14 days after discharge from hospital with a creatinine level of 200 mg and severe oedema of both legs. The following pathologic processes explain his deterioration of function:
  A. Renal artery stenosis.
  B. Acute rejection.
  C. Cyclosporin toxicity.
  D. Renal vein thrombosis.
  E. A viral infection.

5.36 A patient receives a live related donor kidney from his brother. He has good initial function but at three months shows a gradually increasing serum creatinine and urea. The following are recommended:
  A. Urgent ultrasonography.
  B. Empiric reduction of cyclosporin.
  C. Biopsy.
  D. Renogram.
  E. Reassurance followed by cystoscopy.

5.37 The following are true of post-transplant lymphoproliferative disease (PTLD):
  A. The majority are Hodgkin's lymphomas.
  B. Extranodal involvement is most common.
  C. The mortality rate is less for PTLD than for lymphomas in the general population.
  D. It has a high association with the Epstein–Barr Virus.
  E. It may respond to drastic reduction of immunosuppression and antiviral chemotherapy.

5.38 Post-transplant infection is best reduced by:
  A. Prophylactic antibiotics.
  B. Avoidance of immunosuppression.
  C. Isolation of patients.
  D. Correction of any foci of sepsis.
  E. Only using young and healthy donors.

5.39 In paediatric transplants patients should have:
A. Prior immunization.
B. Prior haemodialysis.
C. Doppler ultrasound of major blood vessels.
D. A well-matched kidney.
E. None of the above.

5.40 Kidneys taken from cadaver donors need to be adequately preserved to allow cross-matching and transportation to suitable recipients. Preservation is enhanced by:
A. Warm perfusion with lactate solution.
B. Machine preservation.
C. Colloid perfusion.
D. Perfusion with an iso-osmolar solution.
E. Removal and insertion in cold solution.

5.41 Patients in end-stage renal failure awaiting surgery and a general anaesthetic should have the following:
A. Chest X-ray.
B. Electrolytes including a serum potassium.
C. ECG.
D. Evaluation by a cardiologist.
E. Coronary angiography.

5.42 A 40-year-old patient is undergoing a cadaver donor renal transplant. The crucial factors to which the anaesthetist should pay attention include:
A. A good central venous pressure.
B. Antibiotic therapy.
C. Immunosuppression with release of clamps.
D. Epidural analgesia.
E. Good arterial blood pressure.

5.43 Peritoneal dialysis is:
A. Not markedly different in terms of efficacy from haemodialysis over a 24 h period.
B. Not suitable for patients who wish to perform home dialysis.
C. Not favoured in infants or very young children.
D. Favoured in patients with severe cardiovascular disease.
E. Contraindicated in patients with extensive adhesions from abdominal surgery.

5.44 Relative contraindications to dialysis include:
A. Alzheimer's disease.
B. Multi-infarct dementia.
C. Advanced age.
D. Advanced malignancy.
E. Hepatitis C infection.

5.45 Dialysis is indicated in:
A. Uraemic syndrome.
B. Hyperkalaemia.
C. Metabolic acidosis.
D. Fluid overload.
E. Hypothermia.

5.46 Complications of an arteriovenous fistula include:
A. Thrombosis of the AV fistula.
B. Aneurysm and pseudo-aneurysm formation.
C. Oedema and ischaemia of the hand.
D. Congestive cardiac failure.
E. Frequent infections.

5.47 Physiological principles of dialysis include:
A. The greater the concentration difference across the membrane, the greater the diffusion.
B. The greater the molecular weight of the solute, the greater the diffusion.
C. The inverse relationship of membrane thickness to rate of diffusion.
D. The inverse relation of ultrafiltration to the pressure difference across the membrane.
E. The direct relation of rate of ultrafiltration to the ultrafiltration coefficient (KUf) of the membrane.

5.48 Post-transplant surgical complications include:
A. Graft thrombosis.
B. Lymphocoele.
C. Urine leak.
D. Renal artery stenosis.
E. Bladder diverticulosis.

5.49 Cyclosporin-induced nephrotoxicity is mediated by:
A. Dose-related renal vasoconstriction of the afferent arteriole.
B. Increased endothelial nitric oxide production.
C. Interstitial fibrosis.
D. Thrombotic microangiopathy.
E. None of the above.

5.50 Side effects of azathioprine include:
A. Macrocytic anaemia.
B. Osteoporosis.
C. Pancreatitis.
D. Cataracts.
E. Alopecia.

5.51 The adverse effects of cyclosporin include:
A. Nephrotoxicity.
B. Hirsutism.
C. Gingival hypertrophy.
D. Tremors.
E. Myopathy.

5.52 OKT3:
A. Is an IgG immunoglobulin.
B. Reacts only with human B-cells.
C. Blocks the function of killer T-cells in the allograft.
D. Can cause severe pulmonary oedema.
E. Rarely causes a febrile illness on first administration.

5.53 The following are true of transplant rejection:
A. Hyperacute rejection is mediated by preformed cytotoxic antibodies.
B. It is an infrequent event if the pretransplant crossmatch is positive.
C. Acute rejection is usually cell mediated.
D. Acute rejection can be antibody mediated.
E. Chronic rejection can occur years after transplantation.

5.54 Patients on peritoneal dialysis are prone to:
A. A higher incidence of abdominal wall hernias.
B. Develop sclerosing peritonitis.
C. A higher incidence of diverticular disease.
D. Low back pain.
E. Ischaemic bowel disease.

5.55 Manifestations of post-transplant skin disease include:
  A. Kaposi's sarcoma.
  B. Human papilloma virus (HPV) viral warts on extremities.
  C. Condyloma accuminata.
  D. Fungal skin infections.
  E. None of the above.

5.56 Cytomegalovirus infections can present as:
  A. Pneumonitis.
  B. Oesophagitis.
  C. Retinitis.
  D. Hepatitis.
  E. Cholecystitis.

Locomotor system

1.1   **A.** True
    B. True
    C. True
    D. False
    E. True

Morning stiffness is one of the commonest early symptoms of RA. Ulnar deviation of the fingers at the metacarpo-phalangeal (MCP) joints is generally the result of gravity and the 'Z' deformity of the hand is secondary to radial deviation of the wrist. Rheumatoid factor is generally, but not exclusively, positive. It is the extensor tendons that rupture; flexor tendon ruptures are relatively unusual. Instability at the atlanto-axial level can result in cervical myelopathy.

1.2   **A.** False
    B. False
    C. False
    D. False
    E. False

The ulnar deviation occurs at the MCP joints. The proximal interphalangeal (PIP) joints are prone to develop boutonnière deformities. Synovial hypertrophy is frequent and is generally obvious clinically. RA causes volar (palmar) subluxation of the MCP joints, not dorsal subluxation. Osteoarthritis causes varus deformity; RA causes valgus at the knee. The subcutaneous nodules generally arise on the extensor aspects of the limbs.

1.3 **A.** True
B. True
C. False
D. False
E. False

Rheumatoid arthritis is a systemic disease. It is essentially a disease of the synovium with late bone changes. It mainly affects the MCP joints of the hand leading to ulnar and volar subluxation. Upper motor neurone lesions (UMNL) may result from cervical cord compression at C1/C2. Deformity is common in this disease – arthritis mutilans.

1.4 **A.** False
B. True
C. False
D. True
E. True

The anaemia is generally normochromic and normocytic. Splenomegaly associated with rheumatoid arthritis is known as Felty syndrome. Nail pitting is a feature of psoriatic arthropathy. Pericarditis is frequent but may be asymptomatic. Vasculitis usually affects small vessels and results in haemorrhages or infarcts, often seen in the nail bed.

1.5 **A.** True
B. True
C. True
D. True
E. False

The pathological features of rheumatoid arthritis include (a) synovial proliferation; (b) enzyme production in the articular cartilage leading to chondrocyte destruction; (c) ligament contractures; (d) synovial fluid rich in proteolytic enzymes; and (e) frequent rupture of the finger extensor tendons.

1.6 **A.** True
    B. True
    C. False
    D. False
    E. True

Carpal tunnel syndrome (CTS) is associated with diabetes, which also results in a mononeuritis. Rheumatoid arthritis often causes synovitis that takes up space in the carpal tunnel. Supracondylar fractures result in high median nerve lesions not CTS. Thoracic outlet syndrome usually affects the T1 root and causes wasting of the small muscles of the hand. CTS is associated with acromegaly.

1.7 **A.** True
    B. False
    C. False
    D. True
    E. False

Dupuytren's disaease is not a result of tendon contracture and is solely the result of thickening of the palmar aponeurosis. It has a familial tendency – the curse of the McCrimmonds – but is not caused by an autosomal dominant gene. Diabetes may be associated with carpal tunnel syndrome but not with Dupuytren's. There is an association with both liver disease and use of antiepileptic medication. It is more common in men.

1.8 **A.** True
    B. False
    C. False
    D. True
    E. False

Flexion contractures of the MCP/PIP joints are the usual manifestation of Dupuytren's disease. It is not associated with rheumatoid arthritis nor with gout, but interestingly allopurinol (an antigout medication) is used to minimize its recurrence. Raynaud's phenomenon may be associated with scleroderma that is a cause of PIP joint contracture, but not with Dupuytren's. It is associated with the use of vibrating tools.

1.9 **A.** False
     B. False
     C. False
     D. True
     E. False

The deformity is a result of the contracture of the palmar aponeurosis alone although this may in turn involve both the skin and tendon sheaths, but never the flexor tendons themselves. Skin pits and nodules are the result of extensions from the palmar aponeurosis. The palmaris longus continues into the palmar aponeurosis but is not itself involved. Contracture of the intrinsic muscles leads to flexion of the MCP joints and extension of the PIP joints – the so-called intrinsic plus appearances.

1.10 **A.** True
     B. True
     C. False
     D. False
     E. True

Late infection of total hip replacement is generally the result of metastatic spread from a distant focus of infection. Aseptic loosening is probably the commonest late complication. Dislocation generally occurs within the first six weeks and not usually later. Deep venous thrombosis and pulmonary embolism are early complications. Periprosthetic fracture may occur, especially when associated with loosening of the femoral component.

1.11 **A.** True
    B. True
    C. False
    D. False
    E. True

In osteomalacia, there is either inadequate intake or failure to absorb calcium resulting in reduced serum calcium. The urinary calcium is low as the body tries to retain calcium. Phosphate levels tend to be low as a result of increased bone turnover. Serum alkaline phosphatase is raised reflecting increased bone turnover. The trabeculae are thin with inadequate mineralization of the matrix and increased osteoblastic activity. The bone scan shows generalized increased activity in the long bones reflecting the level of bone activity.

1.12 **A.** True
    B. True
    C. True
    D. True
    E. True
    F. True

In osteoporosis, the bone itself is essentially normal but the volume is reduced. This can be the result of prolonged corticosteroid exposure either therapeutically or through Cushing syndrome. The characteristic radiographic features are of decreased bone density and thin cortices. Bone loss is accelerated after the menopause and may be slowed down by hormone replacement therapy. Vertebral fractures may be asymptomatic and result in the so-called 'dowager's hump' (thoracic kyphosis). Calcium/Vitamin D supplements undoubtedly play a role.

1.13 A. False
  B. False
  C. True
  D. False
  E. False

When standing with the knees locked in full extension the knee is locked in slight hyperextension and so the rectus femoris is not contracted. The popliteus serves to unlock the knee by its action of externally rotating the tibia and is not contracted until then. Not only is the posterior capsule tight but so are the collateral ligaments and the anterior cruciate ligament. The knee can be passively locked in extension but relies on intact femoral nerve function as soon as it becomes unlocked.

1.14 A. False
  B. True
  C. False
  D. True
  E. True
  F. True

Congenital dislocation of the hip is more frequent in girls, and also the firstborn. It is usually picked up in the neonatal period but there are undoubtedly a few cases which present late and are only apparent when the child starts to walk; it may be apparent when the child begins walking but does not cause a delay in walking. The ossification centre appears later and is smaller than the normal side. CDH results in classical true shortening of the leg.

1.15 A. False
    B. True
    C. False
    D. True
    E. True
    F. False
    G. False

Loss of perianal sensation, urinary retention and loss of anal tone are associated with a large disc protrusion which may occlude the spinal canal – cauda equina syndrome. Weakness of ankle dorsiflexion is the characteristic motor finding in L4/5 lesions but ankle plantar flexors receive their innervation mainly from S1. There is also weakness of the extensor hallucis longus. The ankle reflex is S1 mediated and the knee reflex is L3/4. The lateral border of the foot is served by S1.

1.16 A. False
    B. True
    C. False
    D. False
    E. True
    F. True

Avascular necrosis (AVN) of the head of the femur is not associated with gout, which may result in premature arthritis. Gaucher's disease, an inborn error of glucocerebrosidase metabolism, results in alteration of blood flow to the femoral head, and can lead to AVN. The hip is seldom affected in haemophilia. Diabetes has no effect on the vascularity of the femoral head. Deep-sea diving can cause AVN, possibly as a result of gas emboli – Caisson disease. It is also seen in tunnellers. Long-term steroid therapy may cause AVN and is especially seen following organ transplantation and the use of steroids for cerebral malignancy.

1.17 **A.** False
B. True
C. True
D. False
E. True
F. True
G. False

Periarticular osteoporosis is usually seen in rheumatoid disease as are periarticular erosions, which are typical of the synovial proliferation of rheumatoid arthritis. OA causes loss of joint spaces, erosions (which may be seen in both osteo- and rheumatoid arthritis), subchondral cysts (which possibly result from synovial fluid being forced through defects in the articular cartilage into the underlying bone), and osteophytes, which are rarely seen in rheumatoid disease. Soft-tissue swelling is usually the result of synovitis.

1.18 **A.** True
B. True
C. False
D. True

Primary hyperparathyroidism usually results in raised serum calcium and raised alkaline phosphatase caused by increased osteoclastic activity and increased absorption of calcium from the gut. Serum phosphate tends to be reduced as a consequence of increased phosphate loss via the kidneys. Raised urinary calcium often leads to stones in the renal tract.

1.19 **A.** True
B. True
C. True
D. False
E. False

Pathological fractures may result from excessive bone resorption or occasionally through a cyst (brown tumour). Peptic ulceration and pancreatitis are secondary to the hypercalcaemia. Both muscle weakness and reduction of muscle tone may be present. Muscle tetany is a characteristic feature of hypocalcaemia, which is not found here.

1.20 A. False
   B. True
   C. False
   D. False
   E. True

The one and a half medial fingers are innervated by the ulnar nerve. The radial three and a half fingers are innervated by the median nerve. The first dorsal interosseus muscle is ulnar innervated. The abductor digiti minimi is also ulnar innervated. The median nerve innervates the thenar muscles. Nerve conduction studies may be normal in the early stages, especially when the only symptoms are of paraesthesia.

1.21 A. False
   B. False
   C. False
   D. True
   E. True

Haemophilia A has a sex-linked recessive inheritance pattern. Haemophilia B is caused by Factor IX deficiency, and Haemophilia A is a deficiency of Factor VIII. It most commonly affects the knee, elbow and ankle. The clotting time is prolonged but the prothrombin time is normal in Haemophilia A. Osteoarthritis of the ankle generally presents in the fourth decade of life.

1.22 A. True
   B. True
   C. True
   D. True
   E. False
   F. False

In sickle-cell disease, abnormal haemoglobin synthesis results in fragile sickle cells. The anaemia is secondary to the short lifespan of the red cells. Avascular necrosis of the hip results from sludging of the cells in the femoral head. It is also associated with unusual infections especially *Salmonella osteomyelitis*. Steroids may well exacerbate the symptoms rather than relieve them. Bone infarcts are both common and very painful.

1.23 A. True
B. True
C. False
D. False

Neurapraxia results in a transient conduction block, usually secondary to crushing or stretching of the nerve. Neurotmesis involves complete transection of the nerve. Axonotmesis is the result of damage to the axons but the overall architecture of the nerve is intact. Nerves regenerate at the rate of approximately 1 mm a day, or 2.5 cm a month.

1.24 A. False
B. True
C. False
D. False
E. False

The deltoid abducts and flexes the arm. The latissimus dorsi rotates the shoulder internally by virtue of its insertion into the bicipital groove. The pectoralis minor has no action on the shoulder. The serratus anterior protracts the scapula. The infraspinatus abducts and externally rotates the arm.

1.25 A. False
B. True
C. False
D. False
E. True
F. False
G. False

Type II collagen is the main building block of articular cartilage. The collagen and matrix are both produced by chondrocytes. Damaged collagen fibres are repaired very slowly by chondrocytes. The water content of hyaline cartilage is very high. The synovial fluid is the sole source of its nutrition as there is no direct blood supply. There are no nerve fibres in cartilage.

1.26 A. False
   B. True
   C. True
   D. True
   E. True

Developmental (congenital) dislocation of the hip is a clinical diagnosis but ultrasound generally confirms the diagnosis, not technetium scanning. Osteoid osteomata usually demonstrate a typical hot spot on technetium scanning, and any healing fracture will also show up as increased activity. In osteomalacia, there are hot areas classically along the length of the long bones reflecting increased bone activity. Technetium is also commonly used for the diagnosis of bone secondaries.

1.27 A. True
   B. True
   C. False
   D. True
   E. False

The classical Haversian system consists of bone lamellae surrounding a central canal containing osteoblasts and neurovascular bundles. The osteocytes are involved in both bone resorption and formation. Ninety per cent of the intercellular matrix consists of collagen and only 10% water by weight. It also contains hydroxyapatite in the inorganic phase.

1.28 A. False
   B. False
   C. True
   D. True

In tuberculosis, the organism is an acid-fast bacilli. In the UK the human type now predominates. Haematogenous spread is the characteristic mode of dissemination and bloodborne disease infiltrates the joints rather than the diaphyses.

1.29 A. False
   B. True ·
   C. False
   D. True
   E. False
   F. False
   G. True

The ulnar nerve supplies the adductor pollicis, digiti minimi and the hypothenar muscles, and the first dorsal interosseus. The median nerve supplies the abductor pollicis brevis, opponens pollicis and the thenar muscles, and the flexor pollicis muscles.

1.30 A. False
   B. True
   C. False
   D. True
   E. False

In Horner syndrome, the pupil is constricted, there is ptosis, and there is a loss of sweating on the affected side resulting from the absence of sympathetic tone. There is no effect on the occular muscles nor on the cranial nerves responsible for controlling eye movement. Horner syndrome only involves the sympathetic fibres from T1.

1.31 A. True
   B. False
   C. False
   D. False
   E. False

With regard to the anatomical snuffbox, the abductor pollicis longus and extensor pollicis brevis tendons form the more radial boundary, while the tendon of extensor pollicis longus forms the dorsal boundary. The terminal branches of the superficial branch of the radial nerve run superficial to the extensor pollicis longus tendon. The floor comprises the radial styloid and the scaphoid. The radial artery is palpable proximally on the floor of the snuffbox.

1.32 A. False
    B. False
    C. False
    D. True
    E. False

In a tension pneumothorax, the trachea is deviated to the opposite side, the affected side has no breath sounds, the neck veins are distended, and there is hyperresonance on percussion of the affected side. The immediate treatment is by insertion of a wide-bore needle. The chest drain and underwater seal come later.

1.33 A. False
    B. False
    C. True
    D. True

Mandatory radiographs of a severely injured patient include AP chest, AP pelvis and lateral cervical spine. Skull X-rays should be done later and then only depending on the level of consciousness. An AP chest is generally all that is possible. A PA chest requires a co-operative patient who can sit or stand. Lateral cervical spine is important for ensuring that the C7/T1 level is shown.

1.34 A. False
    B. False
    C. False
    D. False

Rapid infusion of 1000 ml is appropriate for an adult but is too great a volume to infuse for children. The fluids should be carefully titrated according to the weight of the child. Twenty-four per cent oxygen is insufficient – aim for 100% which in reality is nearer 85%. There is no indication here to intubate, nor for a DPL.

1.35 A. True
 B. True
 C. False
 D. False
 E. True

Emergency chest drain insertion is needed for an open chest wound, haemothorax and for tension pneumothorax after needle thoracocentesis. Pericardial tamponade should be treated by pericardiocentesis. In a patient with fractured ribs and a flail segment, IPPV may be necessary if there is respiratory distress.

1.36 A. True
 B. True
 C. True

Reduced venous return and secondary reduction in cardiac output may be a cause of patient deterioration after starting ventilation. It is therefore necessary to ensure that fluid replacement has been adequate. It is also important to check that the endotracheal tube is in the correct position. It is also possible to convert a simple pneumothorax into a tension pneumothorax by IPPV. A chest drain may have to be inserted, especially if there are associated rib fractures.

1.37 A. True
 B. False
 C. False
 D. True

Shock is defined as inadequate tissue perfusion. Treatment is aimed at maintaining tissue oxygenation by ensuring adequate intake of oxygen and by maintaining circulating volume. There is no increase in the volume of the third space. Oxygen should be administered at 100%.

1.38 A. True
B. False
C. True
D. False
E. False
F. True
G. False

In pericardial tamponade there is distension of the neck veins as a result of venous congestion. The pulse pressure is narrowed, and pulsus paradoxus is a classical feature. The heart sounds tend to be muffled. The rhythm is unaffected, and the ECG is normal. There is reduced cardiac output leading to a low blood pressure.

1.39 A. False
B. True
C. False
D. False
E. True
F. False
G. False

In Class 2 hypovolaemic shock, the blood loss is 15–30%; the respiratory rate is 20–30. There is delayed capillary return. The pulse pressure is decreased but the systolic blood pressure is normal. The urinary output is 20–30 ml/h. The patient is usually anxious and/or aggressive.

1.40 A. True
B. True
C. True
D. True
E. True

Pulmonary contusions may present with a history of blast exposure. The patient may have chest wall tenderness, progressive hypoxia, haemoptysis and crepitation.

1.41 A. False
B. True
C. True
D. False
E. True

Immediate drainage from a chest tube of >1500 ml is an indication for thoracotomy. Continued drainage of 200 ml/h is likely to indicate significant intrathoracic injury. Pericardial tamponade is usually treated by pericardiocentesis. Thoracotomy should be considered for patients with any sign of cardiac injury, or those who have a large open pneumothorax.

1.42 A. True
B. True
C. True
D. True
E. True

Following a pelvic fracture with disruption of the pelvic ring, all the structures which are closely applied to the pelvis can be disrupted. They include the urethra, the prostate, the bladder, the major blood vessels and the nerves.

1.43 A. True
  B. False
  C. False
  D. True
  E. True
  F. True
  G. True

Urgent referral to a neurosurgical unit should be considered for patients with a deteriorating level of consciousness according to the Glasgow Coma Scale. Disorientation persisting for more than 8 h represents the possibility of a diffuse brain injury. Persistent coma after adequate resuscitation is a neurosurgical emergency but ensure that the patient really is adequately resuscitated and haemodynamically stable. For open skull fractures look for CSF rhinorrhoea, otorrhoea and Battle's sign. Depressed skull fractures may need elevation. Patients with an isolated vault fracture, for example a longitudinal parietal skull fracture, can be observed provided that their condition is stable. Patients with focal neurological signs in the absence of a skull fracture will ultimately require further investigation, but not as a matter of urgency.

1.44 A. False
  B. True
  C. True
  D. True
  E. False

A positive result following diagnostic peritoneal lavage is suggested if there are >100 000 RBC/mm^3, >500 WBC/mm^3, faecal matter in the lavage or a pneumoperitoneum. The presence of urine probably indicates that the catheter has inadvertently entered the bladder – ensure that the patient is catheterized.

1.45 A. False
     B. False
     C. False
     D. False
     E. True

In fractures of the surgical neck of the humerus the axillary nerve may be damaged because it wraps around the surgical neck. The brachial artery, and the radial and median nerves, are further distal to the fracture site. The posterior cord of the brachial plexus is proximal to the axilla.

1.46 A. True
     B. True
     C. True
     D. False
     E. False
     F. True
     G. False

Wrist drop is the classical appearance after division of the radial nerve in the upper arm. All radially innervated extensors will be affected including the extensor carpi radialis longus. Active extension at the MCP joints is by the extensor digitorum comminis which is also affected. The dorsum of the first web space is solely radially innervated and sensation will be lost. Extension at the IP joints is by the intrinsic muscles and remains intact. Opposition of the thumb is median nerve innervated. The first dorsal interosseous muscle is ulnar innervated.

1.47 A. False
     B. True
     C. False
     D. True
     E. False
     F. True

Supracondylar fractures of the humerus in children are often associated with damage to the median nerve, the brachial artery (classically an intimal tear), and Volkmann's ischaemic contracture, which is the classical late complication. Damage to the radial nerve is relatively unusual. The ulnar nerve is generally injured in fractures of the medial epicondyle. The musculocutaneous nerve is more proximal than the fracture site.

1.48 A. True
B. True
C. False
D. False
E. False

In a Colles' fracture, the distal fragment is displaced posteriorly and laterally (radially). The ulnar styloid is also fractured.

1.49 A. True
B. False
C. True
D. True
E. False

The common complications of a Colles' fracture include: (1) malunion, which is one of the commonest complications; (2) carpal tunnel syndrome, especially where there is marked displacement; (3) reflex sympathetic dystrophy (Sudeks atrophy), which is common but unpredictable. Non-union is rare. Rupture of the tendon of extensor pollicis longus is most likely.

1.50 A. True
B. False
C. False
D. False
E. False

The scaphoid is the most frequently fractured of the carpal bones, comprising 80% of carpal bone fractures. It is the proximal pole which develops AVN. Non-union varies from 20–50% depending on the fracture pattern. The major blood supply enters from the distal pole. Displaced fractures of the wrist should be reduced and rigidly fixed.

1.51 A. True
   B. False
   C. True
   D. False
   E. True

Displaced extracapsular fractures of the neck of the femur should be fixed with a dynamic hip screw (DHS) or similar device and not by hemiarthroplasty. The majority of undisplaced intracapsular fractures will heal uneventfully and the risk of avascular necrosis is low. In a 40-year-old with a displaced intracapsular fracture, it is probably worthwhile attempting reduction and fixation to preserve their own joint. A displaced intracapsular fracture in an 80-year-old should be treated by hemiarthroplasty.

1.52 A. False
   B. False
   C. False
   D. True
   E. False
   F. False

Compartment syndrome in the leg also occurs commonly after revascularization. Commonly it is either the anterior or deep posterior compartments which are affected. There is pain on passive dorsiflexion of the toes and loss of sensation over the dorsum of the foot. The dorsalis pedis pulse may well be present. Compartment pressure has to be well over diastolic pressure to confirm compartment syndrome.

1.53 A. True
   B. False
   C. False
   D. True
   E. False
   F. True

A ruptured anterior cruciate ligament is usually accompanied by a 'crack' – often heard by others nearby and felt in the knee at the moment of injury. The effusion, which is a haemarthrosis, is almost immediate. Lachmann's test is negative, and the anterior draw test is positive. It is often associated with the medial collateral ligament and medial meniscus lesions in O'Donoghue's triad. A tibia which sags posteriorly when viewed from the side is suggestive of injury to the posterior cruciate ligament.

1.54 A. False
   B. True
   C. True
   D. True
   E. True
   F. False

The following patterns of tibial shaft fractures are inherently unstable: oblique, spiral, comminuted, and butterfly fractures. Transverse fractures are stable. 'Open' merely refers to the associated soft-tissue injury and is unrelated to the pattern of the bone injury.

1.55 A. False
   B. False
   C. True
   D. False
   E. True

Most midshaft fractures of the clavicle unite without problems. Internal fixation is rarely indicated. The cords of the brachial plexus are related to the subclavian artery and may be damaged. It is the subclavian artery and vein which are at risk, not the axillary. These fractures generally unite within six weeks in an adult.

1.56 A. False
   B. True
   C. False
   D. True
   E. False

Brachioradialis is a weak elbow flexor. Flexor carpi ulnaris flexes the wrist and also causes ulnar deviation. Pronator teres pronates the forearm and is a weak elbow flexor. Flexor digitorum profundus flexes the wrist as well as flexing the MCP, PIP and DIP joints of the fingers. Flexor pollicis brevis is a muscle of the thenar eminence.

1.57 A. True
   B. True
   C. False
   D. False
   E. False

The only way in to the hip via the anterolateral approach is by splitting the gluteal fascia, and passing between gluteus medius and tensor fascia lata. The rectus femoris is not really seen. The sciatic nerve is at equal risk from the two different approaches to the hip.

1.58 A. False
   B. True
   C. True
   D. False
   E. True

The sciatic nerve passes deep to the piriformis. In the posterolateral approach to the hip, the obturator externus and the gemelli are cut to expose the joint capsule. The hip is dislocated by internal rotation and flexion. The sciatic nerve is protected by retracting the short rotators across it. Foot drop/weakness of dorsiflexion are the commonest neurological complications, and are caused by damage to the common peroneal nerve.

1.59 **A.** True
   B. True
   C. False
   D. False
   E. False

A shortened externally rotated leg is the classical presentation of extracapsular fracture neck of femur. With a fracture of the femoral shaft any deformity is possible. Posterior dislocation of the hip causes flexion and internal rotation. Garden grade II fractured neck of femur is by definition undisplaced. Pubic ramus fractures will have no effect on rotation or leg length.

1.60 **1.** E
   2. E
   3. B

Patient 1 should undergo prompt fracture stabilization. Internal fixation of the fracture greatly simplifies subsequent nursing care and may also reduce the incidence of fat embolism, and later of venous thromboembolism. Most femoral shaft fractures are now treated by closed intramedullary nail insertion, that is, without exposing the fracture itself.

Patient 2 has sustained a technically compound fracture of the tibia. Several years ago such injuries were commonly treated by external fixation because of a perceived risk of osteomyelitis. More recently surgeons have tended to treat such injuries with internal fixation, usually intramedullary nailing, as the fracture site need not be exposed during passage of the nail. There does not appear to be a higher risk of infection.

Patient 3 has a complex and comminuted fracture. This type of fracture responds well to skeletal traction, via an os calcis pin, and the talus is gradually drawn distally, allowing the various fracture fragments to fall into place. After a delay of several days, many surgeons will supplement this method with some internal fixation.

1.61 1. D
2. B
3. E

Patient 1 has a considerable soft-tissue defect but has an ideal surface for skin grafting. Muscle and tendon sheath accept split-skin graft readily, and even bone will accept a skin graft as long as the periosteum is intact.

Patient 2 has exposed bone but the amount of tissue loss is not large (around 1 cm² or less) and such an injury will heal by second intention in approximately one month. The exposed bone will gradually be covered by granulation tissue while the skin epithelializes from the edges. If sufficient nail bed is lost (> 50%), then nail regrowth will be disturbed and it is usually better to 'terminalize' the injury, that is, remove the remaining germinal nail bed, trim back the fractured bone end, and close the wound primarily.

Patient 3 will require composite tissue transfer to cover the exposed fracture. Local flaps are not usually possible for distal tibial fractures and a free flap will have to be transferred. Free muscle flaps are usually chosen – latissimus dorsi or rectus abdominis – which are then skin grafted at the same sitting.

1.62 1. B
2. C

Patient 1 clearly sustained a devastating primary brain injury. His level of consciousness has been very low from the outset, and is inconsistent with an expanding intracranial haematoma. His primitive motor responses are highly suggestive of serious intracranial pathology rather than just concussion or the effects of alcohol. Finally his motor responses are symmetrical, as are his pupillary reflexes. This patient has diffuse axonal injury.

Patient 2 demonstrates quite rapid deterioration following injury. She did not sustain a devastating primary brain injury, being able to verbalize at the scene. Her deterioration thereafter is most probably related to a rapidly expanding intracranial haematoma, and extradural haematoma usually appears more rapidly than subdural haematoma. She did not exhibit the classic lucid interval – although many patients with extradural haematoma do not – but demonstrated instead a rapid deterioration in her condition when compared with shortly after the accident.

Vascular system

2.1 **A.** False
   B. False
   C. True
   D. False
   E. False

Carotid stenosis results in ipsilateral amaurosis fugax, as this is caused by platelet/lipid embolism to the ipsilateral ophthalmic artery. Dysarthria, homonymous hemianopia and gait problems are caused by vertebrobasilar insufficiency. Carotid territory symptoms typically include hemisensory and hemimotor signs, amaurosis fugax and loss of higher cortical functions such as dysphasia and visuo-spatial neglect.

   Carotid endarterectomy has been shown to reduce the long-term risk of stroke tenfold in symptomatic patients with severe (> 70%) stenosis. For symptomatic patients with moderate (30–69%) stenosis, carotid endarterectomy offers no additional benefit over aspirin. Carotid endarterectomy has no role in mild (< 30%) stenosis.

2.2 **A.** False
  B. False
  C. True
  D. True
  E. True

The patency rate for superficial femoral artery angioplasty is approximately 60–80% at two years. The technique is ideal for short segment stenosis. As it requires a larger lumen catheter than conventional angiography, the bleeding complication rate is higher. Perforation of the artery can also occur either as a result of the guide wire or through splitting of the calcified plaque. Dissection of the artery can occur but with skill, the guide wire can be made to re-enter the lumen and thus, a subintimal angioplasty can be performed.

Arterial thrombosis can be a complication, particularly in limbs with severe disease and poor run-off.

2.3 **A.** False
  B. True
  C. False
  D. True

Lhermitte's sign describes an acute shock-like pain travelling from the trunk to the limbs. It is caused by cervical spinal pathology such as spondolytic myelopathy and subacute combined degeneration of the cord, but its name is commonly associated with acute exacerbation of multiple sclerosis. Leriche syndrome is the combination of impotence and buttock to calf claudication seen in patients with aortoiliac disease.

Aorto-bifemoral bypass graft has a patency rate of 95% at five years compared to 90% at one year for femoro-femoral bypass graft. However, the latter has a lower mortality rate and is less likely to cause neurogenic impotence. Digital gangrene can occur in aortoiliac disease as a result of showering of microemboli from the ulcerated plaques.

2.4 **A.** True
   B. False
   C. True
   D. False
   E. True

Acute pancreatitis has been reported to cause lower limb ulceration in the form of panniculitis of fat necrosis caused by the effect of circulating lipase. Thyrotoxicosis produces a form of lower leg ulceration called pretibial myxoedema. Ulcerative colitis causes pyoderma gangrenosum of the lower leg.

2.5 **A.** False
   B. True
   C. True
   D. True
   E. True

Typically, venous ulcers are painless and occur predominantly around the medial malleolus (gaiter area) and can extend circumferentially around the ankle. Painful ulcers should raise a suspicion of arterial involvement.

Venous ulcers are caused by chronic venous insufficiency, which may result from reflux of either the superficial and/or the deep venous systems, or obstruction of these venous systems or a combination of both. The absence of varicose veins does not therefore exclude a venous cause of the ulceration.

Chronic venous ulcers exhibit various degrees of lymphoedema, initially pitting but later becoming indurated. the lymphoedema component is initially caused by obstruction of the lymphatics and later by fibrosis through recurrent infection. Chronic venous ulcers can undergo malignant transformation to squamous cell carcinomas (Marjolin's ulcers) in much the same way as chronic sinus is associated with chronic osteomyelitis.

2.6 **A.** True
 B. False
 C. True
 D. True
 E. False

Patients with known atopy such as asthma or a previous
reaction to an iodine-containing contrast medium should be
pretreated with steroid for 48 h prior to angiography to avoid
major reactions. Liver failure is not enhanced by angiography.
Renal function may be affected by contrast medium,
particularly in the presence of renal impairment or heart
failure. Metformin has been reported to cause lactic acidosis
and renal failure following contrast injection. The Royal
College of Radiologists has recommended stopping metformin
for 48 h prior to angiography and not to restart until renal
function has been checked 48 h after it.

2.7 **A.** True
 B. False
 C. True
 D. False
 E. True

Marfan and Ehlers–Danlos syndromes are both associated with
the development of AAA. The association may be linked to
genetic susceptibility through inherited defect in the
structural extracellular matrix or enhanced proteolysis.
Mutations in the type III collagen gene in syphilis rather than
congenital syphilis are associated with the development of
aortitis and aortic aneurysm.

2.8 A. False
  B. True
  C. True
  D. True
  E. True

Ankle ulceration is uncommon in lymphoedema as the skin is more elastic and less liable to be under tension compared to the skin in chronic venous insufficiency. Primary lymphoedema predominately affect young females and is divided into three types: (1) lymphoedema congenita (age <1 year); (2) lymphoedema praecox (age < 35 years); and (3) lymphoedema tarda (age > 35 years). The first two types have a genetic predisposition.

Recurrent cellulitis is associated with lymphoedema as the rapid transport of lymphocytes is delayed in lymphoedematous tissues. The two most commonly involved micro-organisms are *Staphylococcus aureus* and beta-haemolytic Streptococcus.

2.9 A. True
  B. True
  C. True
  D. True
  E. True

Raynaud's phenomenon is seen in connective tissue diseases, most commonly occurring in systemic sclerosis (95%) and mixed connective tissue disease (85%). Other associated conditions include malignancy, drugs (ergotamine, beta-blockers and cyclosporin), occupation (vibration white-finger disease and vinyl chloride disease), thoracic outlet syndrome, cryoglobulinaemia and atherosclerosis (particularly thromboangiitis obliterans).

2.10 A. False
  B. True
  C. False
  D. True
  E. False

The blood is forced through the intima during dissection. Mycotic aneurysms are associated with infection rather than malignancy. Acquired syphilis affects the aorta, the aortic ring to produce aneurysm and regurgitation, and the coronary artery orifices to produce angina. Syphilitic aneurysm usually occurs in the thoracic rather than the abdominal aorta. Mortality from dissecting aneurysm is approximately 50%.

2.11 A. True
  B. False
  C. True
  D. True
  E. True

Diabetics may be unable to feel the pain of ischaemic ulceration because of concurrent sensory neuropathy. Insulin treatment should not be stopped prior to angiography. Diabetics on metformin have been reported to develop renal failure and lactic acidosis after angiography. The Royal College of Radiologists has recommended that metformin should be stopped 48 h prior to angiography and not restarted until renal function has been checked 48 h after the procedure. The most important prognostic indicator of lowering the risk of future amputation is a good control of the blood glucose level.

Diabetics may have calcification of their arteries and thus the ankle brachial pressure index (ABPI) could be over 1 despite the presence of critical ischaemia, as a result of the incompressibility of these calcified arteries. However, the quality of the signal is different from the normal vessel, in that the triphasic signal is replaced by a monophasic damp signal.

2.12 A. True
   B. True
   C. True
   D. True
   E. False

Raynaud's phenomenon usually affects young women.

2.13 A. False
   B. True
   C. True
   D. False
   E. False

Erythema nodosum presents as tender, raised, red lesions usually on the shins but occasionally on the thighs and upper limbs. It is associated with sarcoidosis, Streptococcal infection, tuberculosis, inflammatory bowel disease, Behçet's disease and certain drugs (sulphonamide and penicillin).

Giant cell arteritis affecting the ophthalmic arteries can result in blindness in one or both eyes in 30% of untreated cases. Jaw claudication can occur as well as personality change and angina through the involvement of the cerebral and coronary arteries respectively.

Polymyalgia rheumatica is seen in 50% of cases of giant cell arteritis. Because of this association, the disease is often termed polymyalgia arteritica. Diagnosis is confirmed by temporal biopsy, which shows fibrinoid necrosis with large mononuclear cell infiltrate and giant cells. This process is patchy, however, and is not therefore seen in all cases.

2.14 A. True
   B. False
   C. True
   D. False
   E. True

Buerger's disease is a remitting, relapsing, inflammatory arterial disorder, characterized by thrombosis of the medium-sized vessels. The two main arteries affected are the tibial and radial arteries. It mainly affects male patients and has a strong association with cigarette smoking. When the inflammatory response spreads through to the tunica adventitia, periarticular scarring then causes involvement of adjacent veins and nerves.

117

2.15 A. True
  B. False
  C. True
  D. False
  E. False

Glomus tumour of the nail bed is a benign but painful tumour of the so-called glomus body, which is a highly innervated arteriovenous anastomosis. It has the appearance of a small bluish or reddish raised lesion at the characteristic site of the glomus body. Granulosa cell tumour arises from the ovary.

Kaposi's sarcoma has two components: blood vessels and fibroblasts, the latter showing malignant changes which distinguish it from haemangiosarcoma.

Hamartomata are benign overgrowths of melanocytes. Cholangiocarcinoma is a malignant tumour of the bile duct.

2.16 A. False
  B. False
  C. False
  D. True
  E. False

Subclavian steal syndrome is an uncommon condition characterized by occlusion of the subclavian artery proximal to the origin of the vertebral artery. The patient typically presents with dizziness during excessive use of the affected arm as blood is diverted from the cerebral circulation via the circle of Willis and vertebral artery to the affected subclavian circulation.

2.17 A. False
  B. False
  C. True
  D. True
  E. False

Fallot's tetralogy consists of (1) pulmonary stenosis; (2) ventricular septal defect; (3) overriding of the root of the aorta to the right side of the heart; and (4) right ventricular hypertrophy.

2.18 A. False
   B. True
   C. False
   D. True
   E. False

Early vein graft failure is usually caused by technical or thrombotic problems. Most vein graft failures occur in the intermediate stage (that is, less than two years) as a result of graft stenosis and neointimal hyperplasia. Late vein graft failure is usually caused by progression of the atherosclerotic process.

2.19 A. True
   B. True
   C. True
   D. True
   E. True

Vascular graft infection occurs in between 1 and 4% of cases. Infection should be suspected with recurrent non-specific symptoms such as pyrexia, malaise and lethargy. A chronic wound sinus may also indicate underlying graft infection. Occasionally the wound breaks down with the exposure of the underlying graft. Graft failure may also result from infection.

   Infection of the anastomotic line may lead to false aneurysm formation and in the case of infected proximal aortic graft, this may lead to an aorto-duodenal fistula resulting in catastrophic gastrointestinal haemorrhage.

2.20 A. True
   B. True
   C. True
   D. True
   E. False

True aneurysm of vein graft is rare. It may be associated with structural abnormality not evident at the time of surgery such as varicosity. There is no role for the conservative treatment of false aneurysm as it will eventually lead to rupture or thromboembolism.

2.21 A. False
     B. False
     C. False
     D. True
     E. True

The mechanism of injury in disruption of the thoracic aorta is that of rapid deceleration force. The ascending aorta and arch of aorta are mobile compared to the descending aorta, which is relatively fixed. In rapid deceleration, the shear forces tend to develop in the region just distal to the origin of the left subclavian artery. The majority of patients (over 90%) die before they reach hospital.

2.22 A. False
     B. True
     C. False
     D. False
     E. True

The absolute contraindication to thrombolysis is active internal bleeding. Other contraindications are relative and the risks must be weighed against the benefit of limb salvage.

2.23 A. True
     B. False
     C. True
     D. True
     E. True

Klippel–Trenaunay syndrome is characterized by varicose veins, abnormality of the deep venous system, hypertrophy of soft tissues and bones and haemangiomas (usually the capillary portwine type) of the lower limb. Arteriovenous malformations are usually not present in this syndrome. About 10–20% are associated with digital abnormality but the condition is not hereditary. The condition can affect both legs and other areas such as the pelvis and chest in 20% of cases.

Treatment is usually conservative, with compression bandaging. The deep venous system must be assessed prior to removal of varicose veins as the former is usually abnormal or absent. Complications of this condition include bleeding, venous eczema, venous ulceration, thrombophlebitis, deep venous thrombosis and pulmonary embolism.

2.24 A. False
    B. True
    C. False
    D. True
    E. False

Takayasu's arteritis is an inflammatory and obliterative arteritis primarily affecting the aorta, its branches and the pulmonary artery. The disease affects women more than men with a ratio of 5:1 and has a high incidence in the second and third decades of life. Clinically, it can be divided into two stages. The first is the acute systemic (pre-pulseless) phase characterized by non-specific symptoms such as fatigue, malaise, weight loss and fever. The second is the chronic obliterative (pulseless) phase, the symptoms of which depend on the arteries affected.

Angiography is important as it may show vessel occlusion, stenosis and aneurysmal and collateral formation.

2.25 A. True
    B. False
    C. True
    D. True
    E. True

AAA can mimic symptoms of renal colic, usually with microscopic haematuria. Frank haematuria can occur with aorto-ureteric fistula. The mortality rate from elective AAA repair is about 5%.

Impotence can occur after AAA repair as a result of damage to the autonomic nerves around the aorta and iliac arteries. The incidence is about 1% but the patient must be informed.

Ischaemic bowel can occur after AAA repair as the inferior mesenteric artery is ligated near the sac of the aneurysm. Commonly the distal colon relies on the marginal artery of Drummond and pelvic collaterals for its blood supply after AAA repair.

Those with an AAA have a higher incidence of peripheral aneurysm such as femoral or popliteal. For example, 25% of femoral aneurysms are associated with AAA and 40% of popliteal aneurysms.

2.26 A. False
    B. True
    C. True
    D. False
    E. False

The morphology of the aneurysm is extremely important in endoluminal repair as it should not be too tortuous and there should be enough 'neck' above the aneurysm and below the renal arteries for the stent to lie. Perigraft leakage from the lumbar arteries is specific to endoluminal repair. The natural history is not fully understood but many believe that proximal leaks may predispose to aneurysm expansion and rupture, whereas distal leaks are more benign.

2.27 A. True
    B. True
    C. False
    D. False
    E. True

Leriche syndrome is characterized by bilateral claudication affecting the calves, thighs and buttocks with impotence. The clinical features are caused by the presence of aortoiliac stenosis or occlusion. The condition is usually chronic with the development of collateral circulation supplying the lower limbs despite total aortoiliac occlusion in some cases. The syndrome is not characterized by the presence of carotid stenosis or abdominal aortic aneurysm.

2.28 A. False
    B. False
    C. False
    D. False
    E. True

In woven Dacron grafts, the fabric threads are interlaced in a simple over-and-under pattern, both lengthwise (warp) and circumferentially (weft). Woven grafts have little or no stretch in any direction. They are of low porosity and relatively strong and stiff, thereby reducing the risk of aneurysmal dilatation and elongation. The disadvantages are that they have poorer handling characteristics with a tendency to fray at the edges.

2.29 A. True
   B. True
   C. False
   D. False
   E. True

Diabetic foot disease can be caused by the presence of arteriopathy, neuropathy, infection or any combination of these three processes. Gangrene can occur in a diabetic foot even in the absence of arteriopathy.

Diabetic ulcers usually occur over the pressure points such as the heel or sole of the foot as neuropathy plays an important role – hence the majority of diabetic foot ulcers are usually painless. Venous ulceration typically occurs over the gaiter or malleolar area.

Severe arteriopathy may be present despite a high Doppler pressure. Not uncommonly, the vessels are calcified and become uncompressible when Doppler pressures are performed. As a result, they give a false high reading. Usually these vessels have lost their triphasic flow and become monophasic, which can be detected by the Doppler probe.

A significant proportion of diabetic patients undergo some form of limb amputation. Good control of blood glucose is the most important prognostic factor in these patients.

2.30 A. True
   B. True
   C. True
   D. False
   E. True

Trauma is associated with the development of arteriovenous fistulae. Pregnancy or pelvic mass leads to compression of the pelvic veins and hence venous hypertension. Similarly, deep vein thrombosis causes venous hypertension leading to the development of varicose veins. Leriche syndrome describes the features associated with aortoiliac disease. Klippel–Trenaunay syndrome is characterized by varicose veins, limb hypertrophy and haemangiomas.

2.31 A. False
  B. False
  C. True
  D. False
  E. True

The femoral vein lies medial to the femoral artery. The saphenopopliteal junction is variable in position and should be visualized by preoperative duplex scanning. Saphenopopliteal incompetence is dealt with by ligation of the junction.The Trendelenberg procedure refers to saphenofemoral ligation. Perforator incompetence can be dealt with by endoscopic ligation, so-called SEPS (subfascial endoscopic perforator surgery).

  The present practice for long saphenous varicose veins is to strip the long saphenous vein to below the knee with multiple avulsions. Stripping this to the ankle increases the risk of damage to the saphenous nerve.

2.32 A. True
  B. True
  C. False
  D. True
  E. False

Cervical sympathectomy is indicated for palmar hyperhydrosis, reflex sympathetic dystrophy, small vessel disease and vasculitis. Complications include Horner syndrome, compensatory sweating, gustatory sweating, intercostal neuralgia, pneumothorax and pericapsular pain.

2.33 A. False
  B. True
  C. True
  D. True
  E. True

2.34 A. False
   B. False
   C. False
   D. True
   E. False

Takayasu's arteritis primarily affects the aorta, its branches and the pulmonary artery. Buerger's disease (thromboangiitis obliterans) and giant cell (temporal) arteritis can affect the aorta as well as the large and medium-sized arteries. Polyarteritis nodosa tends to affect larger and medium sized arteries. Wegener's granulomatosis tends to affect medium and small muscular arteries. Rheumatoid arthritis tends to affect small muscular arteries. Allergic vasculitis affects arterioles, capillaries and venules.

2.35 A. True
   B. True
   C. False
   D. True
   E. True

Hypersplenism can result from splenomegaly of any cause. It is commonly seen in portal hypertension, rheumatoid arthritis (Felty syndrome) and lymphoma. It causes pancytopenia and haemolysis as a result of the sequestration and destruction of red cells in the spleen. Treatment is aimed at the underlying cause, but splenectomy is occasionally indicated because of excessive anaemia and thrombocytopenia.

2.36 1. E
    2. G
    3. A
    4. F

Patients with infected grafts usually require an extra-anatomical bypass. In the case of an infected aortic graft, this requires closure of the aortic stump and axillo-bifemoral bypass. Aorto-bifemoral bypass is the procedure of choice for a fit patient with aortoiliac occlusion. Carotid endarterectomy is indicated for patients with symptomatic carotid stenosis in order to reduce the risk of further CVA.

Patients undergoing endovascular repair of AAA with a single lumen graft require femoro-femoral crossover bypass to bring blood to the contralateral leg and ligation of the iliac artery on the contralateral leg.

2.37 1. D
    2. A
    3. F
    4. H
    5. C

Duplex of the carotid is a non-invasive investigation of the underlying cause of TIA/CVA. Venography is a useful investigation for below-knee DVT. For above the knee DVT duplex scan is a non-invasive alternative. An ultrasound scan is the investigation of choice to assess the size of an AAA and also for follow up. It is very much operator dependent.

Doppler pressures are a useful and non-invasive investigation of a patient with peripheral vascular disease. Resting and exercise pressures are useful as the latter often drop in patients with peripheral vascular disease.

2.38 1. B
   2. D
   3. B
   4. E
   5. C

Duplex Doppler scan is the investigation of choice for arterial graft surveillance, for recurrent or atypical varicose veins and for suspected carotid stenosis. Ultrasound scan gives the best measurement of the size of an abdominal aortic aneurysm (AP diameter) but this is operator dependent. Endoluminal aortic aneurysm surgery requires spiral CT scanning to determine the morphology of the aneurysm. MRA or magnetic resonance arteriogram is a useful tool in patients who have severe contrast allergy but it does not give such a high quality of information on distal vessels as a conventional arteriogram.

2.39 1. B
   2. C
   3. E
   4. A
   5. C

Venous ulcers account for about 80% of leg ulceration, 10% of which have an additional arterial element. They typically occur around the gaiter or medial malleolar area and are usually painless and shallow. Two theories have been proposed as to the cause of venous ulceration: (1) the fibrin cuff theory, and (2) the white cell trapping theory. The best conservative treatment is no doubt by graduated elastic compression, which is contraindicated for ulcers with an arterial element.

   Diabetic ulcers are usually caused by neuropathy, ischaemia, infection or any combination of the three.

   Pyoderma gangrenosum has an association, particularly with ulcerative colitis.

2.40 **1.** A
2. F
3. B
4. C
5. D

Panniculitis is an inflammatory condition of the adipose tissues and can be caused by acute pancreatitis as a result of the circulating serum lipase.

Erythema nodosum is a condition where tender, red, raised lesions appear particularly on the shins and less frequently on the thighs and upper limbs. It tends to affect females more than males during the third to sixth decades of life. It is associated with sarcoidosis, streptococcal infection, tuberculosis, inflammatory bowel disease, Behçet's, leprosy and certain drugs such as sulphonamides and penicillin.

Head and neck, endocrine system, and paediatric disorders

Head and neck

3.1 **A.** False
  B. False
  C. False
  D. False
  E. False

Laryngeal tumours most commonly arise in the glottis or supraglottis. Less than 5% occur in the subglottis. They are most commonly caused by cigarette smoke and alcohol consumption. Metastasis is relatively rare. Most laryngeal tumours present with a change to the voice. Stridor is a rare late presentation of either subglottic or supraglottic tumours. Vocal cord palsy may be caused by direct tumour spread into the muscle of the vocal cord or because of involvement of the cricoarytenoid joint. Only a very large laryngeal tumour would cause damage to the recurrent laryngeal nerve because of perineural spread.

3.2 **A.** True
  B. False
  C. True
  D. False
  E. False

Benign paroxysmal vertigo can be associated with head injury. It is also caused by loose particles in the posterior semicircular canal and not the lateral semicircular canal. It may require surgery although this is seldom a treatment. The surgery involves obliteration of the posterior semicircular canal. Stemetil is a central vestibular sedative and is not appropriate for treatment of a peripheral vertigo which is short lived and related to position change only. The standard treatment is Cawthorne–Cooksey head and neck exercises which help with vestibular rehabilitation.

3.3 **A.** True
  B. False
  C. True
  D. False
  E. False

Otitis media with effusion has been associated with parental smoking in children. There is not always a conductive hearing loss particularly if the effusion is small and the mobility of the eardrum is unaffected because there is still a significant amount of air behind it. The eardrum may appear blue if the effusion is longstanding, if it is very thick and tenacious or if it contains a large amount of cholesterol crystals. Most otitis media with effusion will resolve spontaneously and therefore a period of watchful waiting should be employed before surgery. It is non-infective and does not cause facial weakness if left untreated.

3.4 **A.** False
B. False
C. False
D. False
E. False

It is rare to get a CSF leak after nasal trauma. X-ray of the nasal bones is rarely of any benefit. Clinical examination is the most useful examination and X-rays of the nasal bones are not normally recommended. Manipulation of the nasal bones can be done easily up to two or possibly three weeks following the injury; by six weeks the bones would have fully fused. Septal haematoma is a rare consequence of nasal trauma. Epistaxis is normally associated with a compound fracture within the internal nasal cavity and if prolonged requires packing. Cautery will not help as the bleeding is not coming from Little's area.

3.5 **A.** False
B. True
C. True
D. True
E. False

Nasal polyps are associated with late-onset asthma and not atopic asthma, with cystic fibrosis and with aspirin sensitivity particularly with those patients who also have late-onset asthma. Allergic fungal sinusitis may cause massive swelling of sinus mucosa and hence the nasal polyps to appear. People with nasal polyps do not tend to get chronic infective sinusitis nor does chronic infective sinusitis cause nasal polyps.

3.6 **A.** False
B. True
C. True
D. False
E. False

There is no relationship with facial numbness or anosmia, nor with hypernasal speech which is caused by velopalatal insufficiency. Sinusitis is the result of an ascending infection. Nasal regurgitation of fluids is caused by fluid passing through the oroantral fistula.

3.7 **A.** False
B. False
C. True
D. False
E. True

Most CSF otorrhoea will settle spontaneously therefore urgent surgical intervention is not required. Most fractures are longitudinal and so facial palsy is uncommon. Blood behind the eardrum may cause a conductive hearing loss. Fast phase nystagmus to the opposite ear indicates a dead labyrinth of the affected ear and is therefore a poor prognosis. Battle's sign is bruising over the mastoid bone caused by blood tracking from the fracture into the soft tissues over the mastoid and confirms the diagnosis.

3.8 **A.** True
B. False
C. True
D. False
E. False

Lateral rhinotomy is still the classic operation for the excision of inverted papilloma. Nasal polyps are normally removed endoscopically. If they require an open operation this is an external ethmoidectomy. Juvenile angiofibroma can be removed via a lateral rhinotomy or mid-facial degloving approach. Adenoids are removed via the oropharynx. An olfactory neuroblastoma arises within the anterior cranial fossa and would therefore require either a craniofacial resection or an anterior craniotomy to provide exposure.

3.9 A. True
   B. False
   C. True
   D. True
   E. False

Complications of grommet insertion include otorrhoea in
10–20% of patients. There is no reason for dizziness to occur.
A perforation of the eardrum can occur after the grommet
has extruded. Tympanosclerosis is scarring of the eardrum
with deposition of calcium carbonate crystals within its middle
layer and this is frequently seen after grommet insertion.
Grommets are inserted in order to prevent retraction pockets;
there is no evidence that inserting them is a cause.

3.10 A. False
   B. True
   C. True
   D. False
   E. False

Presbyacusis is hearing loss in old age and has no relationship
with objective tinnitus. Glomus jugulare tumour and spasms
of the tensor tympani muscle can produce pulsatile objective
tinnitus heard with an intrameatal microphone. Loud rock
music may cause subjective tinnitus but not objective tinnitus.
Ototoxic drugs, such as gentamicin, may cause subjective
tinnitus but not objective tinnitus.

3.11 A. False
   B. True
   C. True
   D. False
   E. False

Pendred syndrome is usually associated with a goitre but
there is no hypothyroidism. In Usher syndrome there is a loss
of cochlear air cells which are abnormal. Aminoglycoside
deafness is related to a mitochondrial DNA mutation which
makes some patients more susceptible than others to the
effect of aminoglycosides. Profound sensorineural deafness is
usually multi-genetic rather than single gene and is usually
recessive. Most cases of genetically based sensorineural
deafness exhibit a normal cochlea on radiological
investigation.

3.12 A. True
   B. True
   C. True
   D. False
   E. True

Anosmia can be caused by nasal polyps because of blockage of the upper nasal cavity, laryngectomy as a result of air not passing through the nasal cavity, glue sniffing because of damage of the olfactory mucosa, and sinusitis as a result of congestion of the upper nasal cavity causing blockage to the olfactory mucosal area. Epstein–Barr virus does not cause anosmia.

3.13 A. False
   B. False
   C. False
   D. True
   E. False

Ménière's disease normally causes a low frequency fluctuating hearing loss. The tinnitus is subjective and a constant tone. Dizziness lasts for 20–60 min. Pressure can occur in the affected ear. There is no relationship between otalgia and Ménière's disease.

3.14 A. False
   B. False
   C. False
   D. False
   E. False

Pharygeal pouch usually presents with dysphagia or regurgitation of food. It is not premalignant; it is a benign diverticulum. There is no association with gastro-oesophageal reflux. It is caused by a weakness in the posterior pharyngeal wall muscle and does not require surgical treatment if small. Surgical excision is a large operation and should be reserved only for patients in whom endoscopic diverticulectomy has failed and only in those who have large pouches. They are not congenital in origin. They tend to occur in later life.

3.15 **A.** False
   B. True
   C. False
   D. True
   E. False

The only axial flaps are the deltopectoral and nasolabial. Tongue flaps and Abbe–Esslander flaps are local flaps but the pectoralis major flap is a myocutaneous flap.

3.16 **A.** False
   B. True
   C. False
   D. False
   E. True

Vocal cords still move following tracheostomy. There is no speech because air bypasses the vocal cords. Subglottic stenosis is more common in children because the lumen of the trachea is smaller and therefore stenosis is likely to be more significant. Surgical emphysema can occur but it is rare and it is caused by suturing the skin wounds tightly together and then using a tracheotomy tube that is either too small or a cuff that is not properly inflated. In children vertical incision of cartilage is preferred. Indications for tracheostomy include severe respiratory distress.

3.17 A. True
   B. False
   C. False
   D. True
   E. False

T1 and T2 are small tumours and they both have a high cure rate with radiotherapy. T1 is considered to have a 90% cure rate, with 60–70% for T2. T3 describes a carcinoma of the larynx with a fixed vocal cord. Decreased mobility indicates a T2 tumour. When performing a laryngectomy if a collar incision is used then the tracheostomy stoma tends to be made at a separate site. Salivary fistula is a common complication of the surgery resulting from fluid leakage from the pharyngeal repair. T3 NO tumours have no nodes in the neck. There is controversy as to how an NO neck should be treated – as to whether they should be watched or irradiated – but the present guidelines indicate that a prophylactic neck dissection is not required as a part of the treatment.

3.18 A. False
   B. False
   C. True
   D. False
   E. False

A deviated nasal septum is often congenital in origin and is not associated with trauma. Septoplasty and submucosal resection describe a different approach to the surgery to treat a deviated nasal septum and both are valid operations. A deviated nasal septum may cause nasal obstruction which leads to snoring; it is rarely a cause of sinusitis. Many deviated nasal septums are not severe enough to cause nasal obstruction.

3.19 A. False
B. True
C. True
D. True
E. False

Syphilis causes sensorineural deafness. Otosclerosis causes a conductive hearing loss as a result of fixation of the stapes. Otitis externa can cause a conductive hearing loss because of blockage of the ear canal. Tympanosclerosis can cause a conductive hearing loss arising from reduced mobility of the eardrum. Aminoglycoside antibiotics cause a sensorineural deafness.

3.20 A. False
B. False
C. False
D. False
E. False

Topical steroid nasal sprays can be used long term because their action is local and does not occur through systemic absorption. They do not cause rhinitis medicamentosa: this condition is caused by over-use of topical vasorestrictor nose drops, such as ephedrine. Sprays do not need to be used in the head down and forward position: this is only adopted for nose drops. Topical steroid nasal sprays are licensed for the treatment of rhinitis in children.

3.21 A. False
B. False
C. True
D. False
E. True

Neuropraxia has a better prognosis than neurotnmesis, which applies to the death of neurones. Occipitofrontalis is bilaterally represented and is not therefore affected by an upper motor neurone lesion. Electromyography is only useful after degeneration of the neurone and this is not present in the first three days. Parotid malignancy cannot affect Schirmer's test which is testing the function of the greater superficial petrosal nerve which leaves the facial nerve within the temporal bone. Vesicles within the ear can suggest Ramsay–Hunt syndrome caused by herpes zoster virus.

137

3.22 A. False
    B. False
    C. True
    D. False
    E. False

Otitis externa is usually pain free and bacterial. Only rarely are fungal spores seen. The main treatment is aural toilet, that is, cleansing the ear canal and removing debris. Malignant otitis externa is a term used for a spreading infection along the tongue and the skullbase, but it is not malignant and cannot metastasize. There is no relationship between otitis externa and cholesteatoma – the latter occurs within the middle ear.

3.23 A. False
    B. False
    C. True
    D. True
    E. True

The position of the left recurrent laryngeal nerve is variable in its association with the inferior thyroid artery. It is not always anterior and in fact is more frequently posterior. Most retrosternal goitres can be removed without thoracotomy. The superior laryngeal nerve can be damaged dividing the superior pedicle. Thyrotoxic crisis can be prevented by using beta-blockers. Methylene blue can be helpful in defining parathyroid tissue which takes up the methylene blue stain.

3.24 A. False
    B. False
    C. False
    D. True
    E. False

Otitis media with effusion can cause temporary deafness. It is more common in children. There is no discharge because the eardrum is intact. Rhinne's test is usually bone better than air conduction. Cholesteatoma is not a frequent complication but may rarely occur with the development of significant posterior or attic retraction pockets.

3.25 A. False
 B. True
 C. True
 D. False
 E. True

Drooling is caused by poor lip closure and poor control of the tongue. Tonsillectomy alone will not cure it. Tonsils are sometimes removed prior to submandibular duct transposition so that the ducts can be transposed behind the anterior tonsillar pillar. The main indication for tonsillectomy is recurrent tonsillitis. Sleep apnoea in children may be caused by large tonsils causing oropharyngeal obstruction. There is no relationship between cleft palate and tonsil size or frequency of tonsillitis. After removal of the tonsil the parapharyngeal space can be approached, for example, to ablate the glossopharyngeal nerve or to remove an enlongated styloid process.

3.26 A. True
 B. True
 C. True
 D. True
 E. False

Ludwig's angina is frequently caused by dental infection spreading either via the tooth root or via soft-tissue planes into the floor of the mouth. Anaerobic bacteria are not infrequent and hence the need to use an antibiotic that covers anaerobes, such as metronidazole. Massive infection of the floor of the mouth will cause elevation of the tongue base which may compromise the oropharyngeal airway and cause respiratory distress. Ultrasound can help define the tissue space in which the infection occurs and also confirm whether or not there is an abscess present. There is normally an overwhelming infection and this requires treatment with i.v. antibiotics.

3.27 A. False
B. False
C. False
D. True
E. False

Nasal polyps nearly always arise from the ethmoid sinus. They do not tend to occur in patients with allergic rhinitis or hayfever and skin tests are often negative. Nasal polyps usually present lateral to the middle turbinate in the middle meatus having arisen from the ethmoid air cells. Unilateral polyps should always be excised in order to exclude a malignancy. Long-term use of topical steroid nasal drops, such as beclomethasone, should be avoided because of the possible risk of systemic absorption.

3.28 A. False
B. False
C. False
D. False
E. False

Cholesteatoma may form with a marginal perforation and this is therefore an unsafe type of perforation. Many perforations require no surgical treatment because they cause only minimal symptoms. Furthermore, some perforations will spontaneously resolve. Topical antibiotic eardrops can be used with an ear perforation if there is an infection but care should be taken with aminoglycoside antibiotics. Posterior perforations present a greater degree of hearing loss as a result of the round-window baffle effect. The Weber test lateralizes to the affected ear because there is a small conductive hearing loss in the ear with the perforation.

3.29 A. True
    B. True
    C. True
    D. False
    E. False

Snoring patients can present with day-time sleepiness as a result of disturbed sleep patterns because of snoring. Epworth scores are useful in predicting the degree of snoring and the possibility of obstructive sleep apnoea. Palatal surgery can interfere with long-term use of nasal CPAP because palatal escape of air can occur. Snoring is most likely to be caused by palatal flutter rather than by hypopharyngeal collapse. There is no relationship between hyperthyroidism and snoring but there may be a connection with hypothyroidism, particularly if there has been significant weight gain.

3.30 A. False
    B. False
    C. False
    D. False
    E. True

Branchial cysts tend to occur in teenagers or young adults. They tend to be unilateral, presenting anterior to the sternomastoid muscle. They are epithelial cysts and are not premalignant. Association with tracks passing between the carotid bifurcation relating to second branchial arch epithelial cell nests is known.

3.31 A. True
    B. True
    C. False
    D. True
    E. True

Causes of an oroantral fistula include carcinoma eroding the bone and injury penetrating the palate or the anterior wall of the maxilla. Intranasal antrostomy involves surgery between the lateral wall of the nose and the maxillary antrum and cannot cause an oroantral fistula. Surgical ligation of the internal maxillary artery is done via a sublabial antrostomy and if the wound fails to heal a fistula may occur. Dental extraction of premolar and molar upper jaw tooth roots may leave a hole between mouth and maxillary antra.

3.32 A. True
    B. False
    C. False
    D. True
    E. False

Malleus – first arch.
Stapes – second arch.
Styloid process – second arch.
Mandible – first arch.
Thyroid gland – third or fourth arch.

3.33 A. False
    B. True
    C. True
    D. False
    E. True

Goldenhar syndrome is probably the result of multiple gene abnormalities. Treacher–Collins syndrome is caused by autosomal dominant single gene, and Usher syndrome by an autosomal recessive single gene. CHARGE association is probably multiply genetic in origin. Osler's disease is single-gene autosomal dominant.

3.34 A. False
    B. False
    C. False
    D. False
    E. False

All the above may be associated with facial palsy but by definition Bell's palsy is an idiopathic facial palsy. None of these factors can therefore be the cause of a Bell's palsy.

ENDOCRINE

3.35 A. True
  B. False
  C. True
  D. False
  E. False

The thyroid gland normally overlies the 2nd–4th tracheal rings. The superior thyroid artery is a branch of the external carotid, and the inferior thyroid a branch of the thyrocervical trunk.

3.36 A. False
  B. False
  C. True
  D. True
  E. False

Iodide is absorbed from the circulation into the thyroid follicles where it is bound to tyrosine to form monoiodotyrosine and di-iodotyrosine. These then combine to form either thyroxine (T4) or tri-iodothyronine (T3). Thyroglobulin binds thyroxine within the follicles. In serum it Is bound to several proteins including albumin.

3.37 A. True
  B. False
  C. False
  D. False
  E. False

A thyroid nodule is either solitary or part of a multi-nodular colloid goitre. Sudden pain in a nodule may indicate bleeding into a cyst. Investigation with cytology and imaging is necessary to establish a diagnosis.

3.38 A. True
   B. False
   C. True
   D. False
   E. False

Thyroglossal cyst is a remnant of the embryological descent of the thyroid. The thyroid descends from the level of the foramen caecum of the tongue, beyond the hyoid bone to its normal location. Cell nests may occur along this tract, forming a cyst. Classically this is a midline swelling which moves upwards on protrusion of the tongue. Formal excision requires removal of the tract (Sistrunk's operation).

3.39 A. False
   B. True
   C. False
   D. True
   E. False

Hashimoto's thyroiditis results in hypothyroidism. Graves' disease is caused by thyroid-stimulating antibodies. The thyroid gland is very vascular. Other symptoms include tremors, palpitations, weight loss, irritability and restlessness.

3.40 A. True
   B. True
   C. False
   D. True
   E. True

The recurrent laryngeal nerve is a branch of the vagus (Xth cranial nerve) and lies between the oesophagus and trachea, having hooked over the aortic arch on the right and the subclavian artery on the left. It supplies all the muscles of the larynx except the cricothyroid.

3.41 A. False
   B. False
   C. True
   D. True
   E. False

Catecholamines are secreted from the adrenal medulla. The zona glomerulosa secretes mineralocorticoids, the zona fasciculata corticosteroids, and the zona reticulosa the sex steroids.

3.42 A. False
   B. False
   C. True
   D. False
   E. True

These are tumours of the adrenal medulla or related chromaffin tissue and secrete catecholamines. They can occur in the MEN II syndrome with parathyroid hyperplasia and medullary carcinoma of the thyroid. Levels of VMA are raised in the urine.

3.43 A. False
   B. True
   C. False
   D. False
   E. False

Cushing's disease is the excess production of glucocorticoids by the adrenal secondary to a pituitary tumour secreting ACTH. Clinical features of the disease and the syndrome (raised glucocorticoids from other causes) include moon facies, buffalo hump, truncal obesity, muscle wasting, skin pigmentation and diabetes.

3.44 A. True
   B. True
   C. True
   D. True
   E. False

PTH is a polypeptide hormone. Secretion from the parathyroid gland is controlled by negative feedback of high levels of ionized serum calcium. It enhances the formation of dihydroxycholecalciferol, which then increases intestinal absorbtion of calcium. The overall effect of PTH is to raise serum calcium and lower serum phosphate.

3.45 A. True
   B. True
   C. False
   D. True
   E. True

Hyperparathyroidism may be primary, secondary or tertiary. Primary hyperparathyroidism is usually the result of a solitary adenoma, or may be part of a MEN-type syndrome. Secondary hyperparathyroidism occurs because of prolonged hypocalcaemia, most commonly as a result of renal failure. Tertiary hyperparathyroidism can arise as a sequela to secondary hyperparathyroidism where the glands no longer respond appropriately to serum calcium.

3.46 A. True
   B. True
   C. False
   D. False
   E. True

Carcinoid tumours arise from APUD cells (amine precursor uptake decarboxylase) and can occur anywhere along the GI tract. Serotonin is produced, and most lesions occur in the appendix. Ten per cent of patients have liver metastases, and this can give rise to carcinoid syndrome. Raised levels of 5-HIAA are found in the urine.

3.47 A. True
   B. True
   C. True
   D. True
   E. False

MEN I is the association of pituitary, parathyroid and pancreatic islet cell tumour or hormone over-production. MEN II (Sipple syndrome) consists of parathyroid hyperplasia, medullary carcinoma of the thyroid and phaeocytochroma. In MEN IIA, the predominant lesion is medullary carcinoma of the thyroid, and in type IIB, there is associated multiple neuroma and Marfan's features.

3.48 A. True
 B. False
 C. False
 D. True
 E. True

Multiple myeloma causes widespread bone lysis. Medullary carcinomas do not metastasize to bone as commonly as follicular thyroid carcinomas. Bronchial carcinoma can metastasize to bone and produce ectopic PTH.

3.49 A. True
 B. True
 C. False
 D. False
 E. True

Lung, breast, prostate, thyroid and kidney are the most common primary tumours spreading to bone.

3.50 1. B
 2. D
 3. D
 4. B
 5. B

Papillary carcinoma commonly spreads to lymph nodes, and may present with a 'lateral aberrant thyroid'. Histologically, cells with large amounts of cytoplasm are present (Orphan Annie). It tends to occur in a younger population, usually those under 40. Medullary carcinomas originate from the parafollicular or C-cells and occur in association with the MEN IIA syndrome. TSH suppression with thyroxine is important in papillary-type tumours.

PAEDIATRIC DISORDERS

3.51 A. True
   B. False
   C. True
   D. False
   E. True

Oesophageal atresia is a congenital abnormality. It is usually associated with tracheo-oesophageal fistulae. It can cause hydramnios in 60% of cases and also causes premature birth. It is associated with other congenital abnormalities, for example cardiac, bony and other intestinal atresias including imperforate anus.

3.52 A. False
   B. False
   C. True
   D. True
   E. False

In oesophageal atresia, there can be spillage of saliva and intestinal contents into the bronchial tree causing aspiration pneumonitis. It is associated with abnormal development of bones. Tracheo-oesophageal fistulae can be present when the oesophagus is patent and there is no atresia evident. The baby may present with rattling respiration, or with failure to feed and thrive. Delayed diagnosis can increase mortality as a result of complications setting in, such as pneumonitis. Surgery, however, decreases both morbidity and mortality.

3.53 A. True
   B. True
   C. False
   D. False
   E. False

The operation of choice is to perform primary anastomosis of the two oesophageal segments and then to insert a feeding gastrostomy. A two-stage operation where the oesophagus is reconstructed is not commonly performed and is used when primary anastomosis is not possible. Closure of the tracheo-oesophageal fistula is always done. Imaging is important in planning the operation and contrast studies can outline the level of the atresia and of the tracheal communication.

3.54 A. True
   B. True
   C. False
   D. False
   E. False

Pyloric stenosis may present as projectile vomiting and failure to thrive. The pylorus may be felt as a rubbery mass in the right upper quadrant and the strong peristaltic waves of the stomach can sometimes be visible. It is more common in boys with a 5:1 ratio.

3.55 A. False
   B. False
   C. True
   D. True
   E. True

Barium meal used to be the investigation of choice, but ultrasound scan is less invasive and more accurate. The pylorus undergoes hypertrophy, not hyperplasia. This condition may be a genetic disorder but the pattern of inheritance is uncertain. Infants are usually dehydrated and malnourished as they would not have been taking oral fluids for some time and will only have received intravenous feeding after presentation.

3.56 A. False
    B. False
    C. True
    D. True

Metabolic alkalosis is the common biochemical abnormality in pyloric stenosis. Surgery should only be carried out after the biochemical abnormalities have been corrected: the mortality and morbidity of the operation will otherwise be unacceptably high. Ramstedt's procedure is the usual operation and involves the splitting of the pyloric muscles down to the mucosa but without breaching it (pyloromyotomy). If the mucosa is breached, then this is technically a duodenal perforation.

3.57 A. False
    B. True
    C. False
    D. False

Balloon dilation of the pylorus is not a recommended treatment option because in most cases the stenosis recurs. There is still a risk of recurrence after surgery but this is relatively small. Feeding can usually start 8–10 h after the operation. The pyloromyotomy should include about 1 cm of gastric wall as this lessens the risk of recurrences.

3.58 A. True
    B. True
    C. True
    D. False

3.59 A. True
  B. False
  C. False
  D. False
  E. True

In Hirschsprung's disease, the anal canal is always involved with a variable distance of rectum and colon also being affected. The sigmoid is also usually involved but the disease can affect as far proximal as the ascending colon. The myenteric plexus ganglion cells are missing in the diseased segments of bowel. It is a common cause of intestinal obstruction in the newborn, not in older children. It is more common in males than females. Barium enema is possible and will show that the distal colon is narrow. Rectal biopsy is essential to confirm the diagnosis histologically. Treatment can be by formation of colostomy initially to decompress the bowel; more definitive surgery such as rectosigmoid resection and low anastomosis can be performed when the patient is able to undergo major surgery.

3.60 A. True
  B. True
  C. False
  D. True
  E. True

Meconium ileus is associated with cystic fibrosis, which causes thickening of the intestinal secretions and hence a plug of material which gets impacted, usually at the distal ileum. This causes a mechanical obstruction. Contrast enema will show a collapsed colon as this has not been used. Treatment includes the formation of a colostomy and the removal of the impacted material.

3.61 A. True
   B. False
   C. False
   D. True
   E. True

Neonatal volvulus is associated with congenital malrotation of the bowel. The caecum is commonly involved and not the sigmoid. Malrotation causes the different segments of bowel to be fixed at the wrong location and other segments to be free of attachment to the retroperitoneum. This allows the bowel to twist with ease. Ladd's bands can cross the duodenum and when tightened these can cause obstruction. Surgery is required to untwist the bowel and relieve the ischaemia and for inappropriate peritoneal reflections to be divided.

3.62 A. False
   B. False
   C. True
   D. True
   E. True

The defects in an imperforate anus are mainly in the rectum in males, and in the anal canal in females. The defects do not occur proximal to the rectum. Rectovaginal or rectourethral fistulae may be present. The rectum passes through the levator ani muscles especially the puborectalis, and they are important landmarks because those with anal defects arising below these muscles do not need sphincter reconstruction.

3.63 A. True
   B. True
   C. False
   D. True
   E. False

Exomphalos is herniation of the abdominal contents – including the liver – through the base of the umbilical cord. There is usually a covering membrane but this may have ruptured at delivery. It is associated with bowel malrotation and also with other abnormalities especially of the heart. If the defect is small then it should be repaired surgically. It is vital to provide cover for the hernia.

3.64 **A.** True
  B. False
  C. False
  D. True
  E. True

In gastroschisis, the abdominal contents are spilled out via a defect which is usually small and near to the umbilicus but not through it. This is not covered with a membrane and thus the risk of dehydration and infection is high. Surgical repair is usually needed to close the defect and to allow cover for the extruded abdominal contents. It is much less common to find abnormalities of other organs associated with this condition than with exomphalos.

3.65 **A.** True
  B. False
  C. False
  D. True
  E. True

The normal umbilical defect closes soon after birth, usually within the first few days of life. If it remains open, and peritoneum and bowel enter, then it is defined as a hernia. Most of them close eventually by the age of three and therefore any decision on corrective surgery should be delayed until then. They rarely cause obstruction and waiting for the defect to close spontaneously is safe.

3.66 **A.** False
  B. True
  C. True
  D. True
  E. False

Intussusception is a rare cause of abdominal pain in children. The apex of the intussusception may be formed by polyps, Meckel's diverticulum, or swollen and inflamed lymphoid tissue. The lead point is usually at the distal ileum and progresses to involve the terminal ileum. Males are much more commonly affected than females.

3.67 A. True
 B. False
 C. True
 D. False
 E. False

In intussusception, the common symptom is colicky abdominal pain. Vomiting may be present but is not projectile in nature (pyloric stenosis). The affected segment is usually palpable as a sausage-shaped mass in the right side of the abdomen. Redcurrant-coloured stool which is like jelly may be passed and is characteristic of this condition. The abdomen is not scaphoid in appearance, and may be distended as a result of intestinal obstruction.

3.68 A. False
 B. True
 C. False
 D. True
 E. False

In intussusception, plain X-rays are not contraindicated, but they may not be helpful in the diagnosis. Barium enema is the most useful diagnostic test and the intussusception may also be reduced under the hydrostatic pressure of the column of barium. This conservative method of reduction should be tried initially. If this is unsuccessful, surgical reduction will be needed and the affected segment may have to be resected if reduction is not possible.

3.69 A. False
 B. True
 C. False
 D. True
 E. False

3.70 A. False
   B. True
   C. False
   D. True
   E. False

Meckel's diverticulum is present in about 2% of the population, found about 60 cm from the terminal ileum, and about 5 cm long. It is a remnant of the vitello-intestinal duct and often contains ectopic pancreatic and gastric tissue. The ectopic gastric tissue can cause peptic ulcers, and haemorrhage is the most common complication and presenting complaint. However it is not present in all cases. When inflamed, it may cause abdominal pain and can mimic acute appendicitis. Technetium scan is most useful if the diverticulum contains gastric mucosa, as the take-up is high in these cells. Barium meal is not useful. The diverticulum which is found incidentally should not be excised if it does not look inflamed.

3.71 A. False
   B. False
   C. False
   D. False
   E. False

Wilm's tumour is a nephroblastoma. Fetal neural crest cells are involved in the formation of neuroblastomas. Wilm's tumours usually present as an abdominal mass in children up to five years old. CT scanning is most useful for assessing the size and extent of the tumour; selective angiography is unhelpful. Excision of the tumour is always performed, and chemo- and radiotherapy are only given to certain patients.

3.72 A. True
B. False
C. False
D. True
E. True

Torsion of the testicle is a surgical emergency as the testicle will undergo infarction after 6 h of ischaemia. It most commonly presents with testicular pain but may present just with abdominal signs. It is not caused by torsion of the hydatid of Morgagni nor of any other testicular appendage. It is not caused by epididymo-orchitis. At surgery, the unaffected side should always be fixed to the scrotum to prevent that testicle undergoing torsion at a later date.

3.73 A. True
B. False
C. True
D. True
E. False

Congenital inguinal hernia is caused by a patent processus vaginalis and may be bilateral. The defect may close naturally during the first year of life and thus surgery should be delayed until at least the second year. The hernia sac should be tied off at the deep inguinal. There is no need for repair of the abdominal wall as this is normal.

3.74 A. True
B. True
C. True
D. False
E. True

In congenital diaphragmatic hernia, neonates usually present with respiratory distress, displaced apex beat and scaphoid abdomen. The defect is commonly in the posterolateral position of the left side. Intubation and ventilation should be started as soon as the diagnosis is made and the decision taken to operate. Pulmonary hypoplasia may be present and is caused by the lack of space for development.

3.75 A. False
  B. True
  C. True
  D. True

The daily requirement of neonates for water is 100–150 ml/kg; for amino acid it is 2 g/kg; and calorie intake should be 100 kcal/kg. The minimum urine output should be 1 ml/kg/h.

3.76 1. F
  2. C
  3. B

Pneumonia will present with respiratory distress but the other histories and signs make this an unlikely diagnosis in each of these scenarios. Diaphragmatic hernia can present with a scaphoid abdomen as its contents are in the chest cavity. This causes the lungs to develop and expand poorly, leading to respiratory distress. In oesophageal atresia, mucus produced in the intestinal tract is often in communication with the trachea and this causes noisy breathing with frothing. In cystic fibrosis, the mucus is thick and difficult to expel but the associated respiratory problems do not usually present so soon after birth. In Fallot's tetralogy, the baby is cyanosed as a result of the shunting of oxygenated blood, and respiratory distress is not a main presenting feature. In choanal atresia, there is no air entry through the nose and babies are obligatory nasal breathers. This is why forced oral breathing while crying brings air into the lungs and relieves the cyanosis.

3.77 1. B
2. C
3. F

Meckel's diverticulum commonly presents with gastrointestinal haemorrhage and abdominal pain, not vomiting. In pyloric stenosis, male children aged 3–6 weeks present with projectile vomiting and failure to thrive. The hypertrophied pylorus may be palpable in the upper abdomen. Duodenal atresia is associated with Down syndrome and the child presents with vomiting and a double bubble on the erect film, which represents air in the stomach and in the duodenum, proximal to the obstruction. Intussusception presents with severe colicky abdominal pain and vomiting may be present. The affected segment may be palpable as a sausage-shaped mass.

Diaphragmatic hernia presents with respiratory distress. Meconium ileus is associated with cystic fibrosis, and the thick plug of meconium can become impacted in the terminal ileum causing small bowel obstruction.

Abdomen

4.1   **A.** False
     B. True
     D. True
     D. True
     E. False

Congenital inguinal hernias rarely strangulate and usually reduce spontaneously with analgesia or with gentle manipulation. Direct inguinal hernias are more common in patients who have undergone appendicectomy because damage to the ilioinguinal nerve which supplies the conjoint tendon may occur with a Lanz or Grid iron incision. Although unusual, a right inguinal hernia may contain the sigmoid colon but the small intestine is more common with a tendency to strangulation. Littre's hernia contains a Meckel's diverticulum.

4.2   **A.** True
     B. True
     C. True
     D. False
     E. True

The formation of an abdominal stoma is associated with clinical depression in 10–30% of cases. Parastomal fistulae may be associated with Crohn's disease, but more commonly are caused by passage of the suture through the mucosa inside the ileostomy. Loop stomata prolapse more frequently than end stomata. High stomal output may lead to hyponatraemia caused by the high sodium content in ileostomy effluent. Ileostomy complications are common, reaching a cumulative rate of more than 50% over ten years, the commonest being parastomal hernia.

4.3 **A.** False
  B. True
  C. False
  D. False
  E. False

The commonest cause of small bowel villus atrophy in the UK is coeliac disease. It usually improves with a gluten-free diet. Although historically the Crosbie capsule was used in the investigation of malabsorption, small bowel biopsies are now obtained endoscopically. Coeliac disease is associated with T-cell lymphoma. There is no known association between coeliac disease and intestinal metaplasia.

4.4 **A.** True
  B. False
  C. False
  D. False
  E. False

Large bowel obstruction may result in small bowel dilatation when there is incompetence of the ileocaecal valve (about 50% of the population). When dilatation is confined to the large bowel, this is termed closed loop obstruction and requires urgent treatment to prevent caecal perforation. Rectal lesions rarely present with obstruction because they cause rectal bleeding and tenesmus which leads the patient to seek medical advice before obstruction develops. Vomiting is a relatively late event in large bowel obstruction but electrolyte imbalance frequently occurs. Pseudo-obstruction cannot be excluded on plain films and an unprepared water-soluble contrast enema should be performed.

4.5 **A.** True
  B. False
  C. False
  D. True
  E. True

Mesenteric venous occlusion classically presents insidiously with abdominal pain over several weeks. Signs may be out of proportion to abdominal signs. The diagnosis is usually made at laparotomy when resection of ischaemic bowel may be required followed by post operative anticoagulation. It is associated with oral contraceptive pills containing oestrogen and with inherited hypercoagulable states.

4.6 **A.** False
    B. False
    C. True
    D. False
    E. False

Low anterior resection does not have a higher incidence of local recurrence than abdominoperineal resection provided that either procedure incorporates total mesorectal excision. The patient is positioned in the Lloyd-Davies position. In the event of damage to the sympathetic nerves, ejaculatory difficulty may occur. Many surgeons will protect a low coloanal anastomosis with a temporary stoma although this is not considered mandatory. At present there is no evidence to suggest that neoadjuvant chemoradiation confers a survival advantage.

4.7 **A.** False
    B. False
    C. True
    D. False

Laparoscopic procedures avoid upper abdominal incisions which may compromise postoperative respiration if pain control is inadequate. However, the intraoperative respiratory compromise exerted by the pneumoperitoneum is likely to make a laparoscopic procedure unsuitable for patients with severe respiratory disease. Laparoscopic cholecystectomy is now frequently performed for acute cholecystitis. Although laparoscopic cholecystectomy is associated with a higher overall incidence of bile duct injury than open cholecystectomy, the incidence of major duct injury is not significantly different. The invasion caused by laparoscopic cholecystectomy is the same as open cholecystectomy, only the access is less.

4.8 **A.** False
  B. False
  C. False
  D. True
  E. True

The predominant blood supply to the stomach is from the coeliac trunk but the right gastroepiploic arises from the superior mesenteric artery. The stomach is derived from the foregut and therefore does not participate in the midgut herniation which occurs during normal development. When the stomach rotates during development the left vagus comes to lie anteriorly and the right vagus posteriorly. B-cell lymphoma occurs more commonly in the stomach than in any other part of the GI tract.

4.9 **A.** False
  B. False
  C. False
  D. False
  E. False

Overall five-year survival in patients with carcinoma of the oesophagus is 10% and is more common in males in the UK. Although tylosis is rare, all patients with the condition develop oesophageal carcinoma. Oesophageal carcinoma does not respond well to chemotherapy and is not known to be associated with high salt intake – although gastric cancer is.

4.10 **A.** False
  B. False
  C. True
  D. True
  E. False

Peptic ulcer disease rarely presents with gastric outlet obstruction in Western countries. It causes metabolic hypochloraemic alkalosis and may present with Trousseau's sign because of hypocalcaemia. Hypocalcaemia develops through low ionized calcium levels in alkalosis. Perforation at ERCP can produce localized abscess causing gastric outlet obstruction. Gastric outlet obstruction occurs in babies as a result of congenital hypertrophic pyloric stenosis.

4.11 A. True
    B. True
    C. True
    D. False
    E. False

The overall mortality of acute pancreatitis is 10%, with 30% for severe pancreatitis. Thiazide diuretics or seatbelt trauma may cause acute pancreatitis. *E. coli* infection is not a common aetiological agent in acute pancreatitis although it may be a complication. There is no relationship between the level of the plasma amylase and the severity of inflammation.

4.12 A. False
    B. True
    C. True
    D. False
    E. True

Linitis plastica rarely causes gastrointestinal bleeding but usually presents with weight loss, poor appetite and early satiety. Intestinal-type gastric carcinoma is classically associated with *Helicobacter pylori* infection rather than the diffuse type (Linitis plastica). It tends to present late and has a poor prognosis. The mucosa is often normal on endoscopy, but reduced gastric distension and peristalsis may be apparent.

4.13 A. False
    B. False
    C. False
    D. False
    E. True

The inguinal canal contains the ilioinguinal nerve. In the neonate the superficial and deep rings overlie one another so that the inguinal canal does not exist. The inguinal canal extends from the deep ring situated at the midpoint of the inguinal ligament to the superficial ring. The mid-inguinal point is the surface marking of the femoral artery. In the female the inguinal canal contains the round ligament of the uterus.

4.14 A. False
    B. True
    C. True
    D. True
    E. False

Faecal incontinence in the elderly is common and is usually the result of faecal impaction secondary to reduced anorectal sensation. Occasionally, rectal cancer may present with faecal leakage. Treatment with a low residue diet to firm the stool and regular suppositories to assist adequate evacuation may be effective. The effects of obstetric injuries may not become apparent until old age. Post-anal repair has very poor long-term results.

4.15 A. False
    B. True
    C. True
    D. True
    E. False

Carcinoid tumours are associated with raised urinary 5-HIAA (hydroxy indole acetic acid). They are characteristically slow growing and may present to respiratory physicians with wheezing and facial flushing; they may be difficult to differentiate from rosacea in the long term. Carcinoid tumours commonly metastasize to the liver but not to the brain.

4.16 A. True
    B. False
    C. False
    D. False
    E. False

Hepatic colorectal metastases are more common in the right lobe and are predominantly supplied by the hepatic artery. They uncommonly present with jaundice. The absolute number of metastases is not a contraindication to surgery; it is the distribution and the volume of functioning liver that would remain after resection that determines operability. They do not respond well to radiotherapy.

4.17 A. False
   B. True
   C. False
   D. False
   E. False

Carcinoma of the gallbladder is a rare cause of GI malignancy and has a very poor prognosis. It is strongly associated with cholesterol gallstones but there is no known association with non-steroidal anti-inflammatory drugs. It is not radiosensitive.

4.18 A. True
   B. True
   C. True
   D. True
   E. False

Stones in the biliary ducts cause an increase in plasma alkaline phosphatase and the oral contraceptive pill can cause intrahepatic cholestasis with an increase in alkaline phosphatase. Sclerosing cholangitis may complicate ulcerative colitis and rising alkaline phosphatase is one of the earliest signs. Alkaline phosphatase is raised in osteomalacia because of increased osteoblastic activity but is normal in osteoporosis.

4.19 A. True
   B. False
   C. True
   D. False
   E. False

After ten years of extensive ulcerative colitis (defined as extending beyond the splenic flexure) the risk of malignancy is 2% per year. Toxic megacolon occurs when an acute colitic becomes toxic (tachycardia, pyrexia, leucocytosis) and colonic dilatation occurs. There is no agreed definition of the degree of dilatation required but 5–6 cm is generally quoted. Toxic megacolon can be treated conservatively in the first instance with intravenous fluids and steroids. Twice-daily clinical examination and daily abdominal X-rays should be performed to reassess the condition of the patient and colon. If there is no substantial improvement or deterioration occurs within 24–48 h then this should be an indication for emergency surgery. Indications for colectomy may be classified as emergency or elective. Emergency indications include acute fulminant colitis, toxic megacolon, perforation or haemorrhage. Elective indications include failure to respond to medical treatment, unacceptable side effects of medication, the development of malignancy or dysplasia, growth failure in children and occasionally extraintestinal manifestations. Emergency surgery involves colectomy and formation of an ileostomy. The rectal stump may be exteriorized as a mucous fistula or oversewn: this allows the patient to recover from the acute event and proctectomy can be performed at a later date. Reconstruction with an ileoanal pouch can then be considered. Smoking appears to protect against ulcerative colitis but to aggravate Crohn's disease.

4.20 A. False
    B. False
    C. False
    D. False
    E. False

Splenectomy for trauma should be avoided wherever possible because of the risk of overwhelming post-splenectomy sepsis. Despite the various techniques described for splenic preservation these are frequently unsuccessful in stopping bleeding. Although the risk of sepsis is higher in children, this does not contraindicate splenectomy if required. Post-splenectomy sepsis is caused by encapsulated bacteria, particularly *Streptococcus pneumoniae* and *Haemophilus influenzae*. Where possible vaccination with pneumovax, HIB vaccine and meningococcal vaccine should be performed preoperatively. Although laparoscopic splenectomy may be possible in the elective situation, it is not to be recommended for trauma.

4.21 A. True
    B. False
    C. True
    D. True
    E. True

Chylous ascites can look milky or cloudy on inspection. It is rare and arises as a result of damage to the intra-abdominal lymphatics or cisterna chyli by blunt trauma, iatrogenic injury during aortic surgery or as a result of obstruction of the lymphatics from pancreatic carcinoma or chronic pancreatitis. It is not a recognized complication of cholecystectomy. Chylous ascites following iatrogenic injury may be treated conservatively or surgically; conservative treatment involves dietary manipulations to reduce the volume of lymph produced, consisting of a diet high in medium-chain fatty acids which can be directly absorbed from the small intestine.

4.22 **A.** False
  B. False
  C. False
  D. True
  E. True

The oesophagus has three layers, mucosa, submucosa and a muscular layer. There is no serosa. It passes through the diaphragm via the oesophageal hiatus at T10 and is crossed by the azygos vein just above the tracheal bifurcation. The blood supply to the oesophagus is from the inferior thyroid artery (from the thyrocervical trunk) in the upper third, from oesophageal branches directly from the aorta in the middle third and from the left gastric artery in the lower third. The incidence of oesophageal atresia is 1:2500 live births.

4.23 **A.** True
  B. False
  C. False
  D. False
  E. True

When severe, gastro-oesophageal reflux disease may cause dental erosions secondary to acidic refluxate. It is very rare in the Asian subcontinent. In infants gastro-oesophageal reflux commonly causes respiratory complications, but this is rare in adults. The severity is graded by De Meesters' scoring system. Bernstein's acid perfusion test can be used to make the diagnosis, although this is rarely used today. It has been replaced by ambulatory pH and manometry and combined with endoscopy.

4.24 A. True
   B. True
   C. True
   D. False
   E. True

Achalasia of the oesophagus is a motility disorder characterized by the failure of relaxation of the lower oesophageal sphincter and absent peristalsis in the oesophageal body. Treatment with Botulinum toxin results in temporary improvement in symptoms. One of the known complications of cardiomyotomy is gastro-oesophageal reflux and for this reason many surgeons combine cardiomyotomy with an antireflux procedure. Chagas' disease – which is a late complication of infection with the South American trypanosome – presents a similar radiological appearance with proximal oesophageal dilatation tapering to a rat's tail.

4.25 A. True
   B. False
   C. False
   D. False
   E. True

Massive lower GI bleeding settles spontaneously to allow full investigation of a stable patient 80–90% of the time. If bleeding continues emergency investigation is required. Colonoscopy in the acute setting rarely identifies the source of bleeding. A radio-labelled red-cell scan requires bleeding at a rate of 0.5 ml/min while angiography requires losses of 1–2 ml/min. The commonest causes of massive colonic bleeding in the elderly are diverticular disease and angiodysplasia.

4.26 A. False
   B. True
   C. True
   D. False
   E. False

Acute acalculus cholecystitis is usually seen in acutely ill patients often in the intensive care unit with multi-organ failure. It is thought to be a result of reduced splanchnic perfusion. Unlike calculus cholecystitis, it is unrelated to gallbladder cancer. Treatment by timely percutaneous cholecystostomy may prevent gangrene or perforation and avoids surgery in otherwise unfit patients.

4.27 A. True
   B. False
   C. True
   D. False
   E. False

Non-surgical treatment of gallstones is accompanied by a very high recurrence rate (90%). Ursodeoxycholic acid may dissolve non-calcified stones but needs to be taken for 18–24 months. It should probably be continued to prevent reformation of stones but this is not favoured by patients who frequently experience severe nausea. Methyl terbutyl ether (MTBE) can be instilled into the bile duct and cause effective stone dissolution. It is not generally recommended for young patients because of its high recurrence rates and patients requiring immunosuppression should generally be treated by cholecystectomy.

4.28 A. True
   B. True
   C. False
   D. False
   E. True

Cholangiocarcinoma is a rare cancer representing 1% of GI cancers. It is predisposed to by choledocholithiasis, sclerosing cholangitis, clonorchis sinensis infection and choledochal cysts. It is a locally invasive cancer which metastasizes late. The prognosis is poor with only 20% of tumours being resectable and a five-year survival of 5–20%.

4.29 A. True
B. False
C. True
D. False
E. True

Sclerosing cholangitis is associated with ulcerative colitis in 70–80% of cases and to a much lesser extent with Crohn's disease. It is commoner in males and the predominant age of onset is 40–50 years. It usually presents with cholestatic jaundice although it may be suggested by an isolated raised alkaline phosphatase in a patient with inflammatory bowel disease. It may rarely present with fulminant hepatic failure. There is diffuse involvement of the whole biliary tree in 80% of cases.

4.30 A. False
B. False
C. True
D. False
E. False

The clotting defect associated with jaundice involves the Vitamin K dependent factors, namely II, VII, IX and X. Correction can be achieved with Vitamin K when over 48 h is available but in the emergency situation fresh frozen plasma is required.

Choledocholithiasis rarely requires emergency surgery; cholangitis is treated medically in the first instance and stones can usually be removed endoscopically. Hepatorenal failure may complicate jaundice and can usually be avoided by maintaining adequate hydration preoperatively.

4.31 A. True
B. False
C. False
D. False
E. True

Adenocarcinoma of the pancreas presents late because of the retroperitoneal position of that organ. The overall five-year survival is 1–2%. It is not known to be related to oral contraceptive usage. The monoclonal tumour marker Ca 19-9 has a sensitivity of 80–90% but low specificity. Pancreatic cancer may rarely present with paraneoplastic phenomena such as peripheral neuropathy.

4.32 A. True
B. False
C. False
D. False
E. True

Gastrinoma results in high gastrin secretion and leads to peptic ulceration. This may be atypical in site, often occurring in the distal duodenum and jejunum. They are malignant in 60–80% of cases. Identification of the site of the tumour can be very difficult because of the small size of tumours and they are frequently located in the duodenal wall. In MEN type II there is no association with pituitary tumours so no explanation for optic chiasm pressure. MEN type I consists of pituitary, pancreatic and parathyroid tumours.

4.33 A. True
B. True
C. False
D. True
E. False

Portal hypertension is most commonly caused by alcoholic cirrhosis in Western societies. Other causes include prehepatic portal vein thrombosis and post-hepatic Budd–Chiari syndrome. Budd–Chiari syndrome is caused by hepatic venous thrombosis and results in caudate lobe hypertrophy. To date, the use of TIPSS has been confined to patients with complicated portal hypertension, that is, bleeding varices. The early mortality from an initial variceal bleed is 50%. Oesophageal transaction is rarely needed today with the use of sclerotherapy, banding and TIPSS. The procedure is performed through a gastrotomy: a circular stapler is inserted into the lower oesophagus and the oesophagus transected and restapled as one procedure.

4.34 A. False
  B. True
  C. True
  D. False
  E. True

Urinary tract infection is rare in young or middle-aged men, so other causes of lower abdominal pain (such as a pelvic appendix causing bladder inflammation) should be considered first. Similarly acute diverticulitis may cause bladder or ureteric inflammation. Exercise-induced microscopic haematuria may occur in young men. Microscopic haematuria in a catheter specimen of urine may be caused by the trauma of catheter insertion.

4.35 A. True
  B. True
  C. True
  D. False
  E. True

An increase in plasma amylase greater than five times normal is generally considered diagnostic of acute pancreatitis provided that the symptoms and signs are compatible. Ischaemic gut can also result in a similar rise in plasma amylase, but this may be suggested from the history, the presence of cardiac arrhythmias, a very high white-cell count and dilated loops of small bowel on X-ray with intramural gas or gas in the portal vein. Other causes of raised plasma amylase include ruptured ectopic pregnancy, ruptured aortic aneurysm, perforated duodenal ulcer, acute parotitis and failure of renal excretion. Infusion of starch-containing colloid fluids also results in raised plasma amylase.

4.36 A. False
　　B. True
　　C. False
　　D. False
　　E. True

Recurrent perianal sepsis may be a result of underlying Crohn's disease, but is much more likely to be caused by a fistula. If culture of pus from a perianal abscess yields skin flora then an underlying fistula is extremely unlikely. If gut organisms are cultured, then this increases the possibility of a fistula. A fistula in ano should not be laid open at the time of abscess drainage as it is difficult to assess the degree of sphincter involvement when the patient is anaesthetized and there is perianal induration. Extrasphincteric fistula is indicative of pelvic sepsis with underlying pathology and this requires investigation and treatment. A loose seton is used to eradicate sepsis, often prior to definitive fistula treatment but it may sometimes be permanent.

4.37 A. False
　　B. True
　　C. True
　　D. False
　　E. True

The symptoms of haemorrhoids arise as a result of abnormalities of the anal vascular cushions. Treatment is conservative and surgical. Conservative treatment includes dietary manipulation, injection sclerotherapy with phenol in oil and rubber-band ligation. Surgical treatment is by excision. In the past lateral internal sphincterotomy has been used in treatment with some success. Thrombosed haemorrhoids may be treated conservatively with analgesia, bed rest and ice packs or by emergency haemorrhoidectomy. There is a theoretical risk of portal pyaemia from the surgery of thrombosed haemorrhoids. Weeping from the perianal wound for up to six weeks after haemorrhoidectomy is normal.

4.38 A. False
  B. True
  C. True
  D. False
  E. True

Parenteral feeding inhibits the adaptation of the small bowel after massive resection. The ileum is better at adaptation and the preservation of the ileocaecal valve is important. More complex substrates produce better adaptation so that addition of some complex carbohydrates is better than elemental diets. Inhibition of adaptation is caused by steroids.

4.39 A. False
  B. True
  C. False
  D. False
  E. False

Femoral hernia is four times as common in women as in men. It emerges below and lateral to the pubic tubercle. Although it may be difficult to differentiate an incarcerated femoral hernia from an inguinal lymph node, metastases from rectal cancer to inguinal nodes are very unusual. Femoral hernias may be repaired by a mesh plug, but no recommendation of this method is made in guidelines. Both femoral hernia and saphena varix have a cough impulse. The saphena varix reduces spontaneously on lying down while the femoral hernia may require manipulation to reduce. The presence of varicose veins also suggests a saphena varix.

4.40 A. True
  B. True
  C. False
  D. True
  E. False

The congenital umbilical hernia is associated with Down syndrome. Strangulation is rare (2%). It commonly closes spontaneously in children under three years but is unlikely to do so in children older than this. Hernias larger than 2 cm in younger children are unlikely to close and should be treated surgically. They do not require mesh, and suture provides adequate repair.

4.41 A. True
    B. True
    C. True
    D. False
    E. False

Differential diagnoses of hernias:

Inguinal hernia	Femoral hernia
Femoral hernia	Inguinal hernia
Vaginal hydrocele	Lymphadenopathy
Hydrocele of cord	Saphena varix
Undescended testis	Ectopic testis
Lipoma of cord	Psoas abscess
	Psoas bursa
	Lipoma

4.42 A. True
    B. True
    C. True
    D. True
    E. False

Inguinal hernias are commoner in premature and low birthweight babies. The ratio is M:F 9:1. Seventy per cent are right sided and 25% are left sided. Five per cent are bilateral. Thirty per cent are present in the first year of life and are caused by the congenital persistence of the ductus vaginalis.

4.43 A. True
    B. False
    C. True
    D. False
    E. True

The F:M is 4:1. It is commonest in middle-aged and elderly women, and is also more common in parous women. They are much less common than inguinal hernias overall, but are as common as inguinal hernias in older women. They appear medial to the femoral vein. They have a higher risk of strangulation. There is often no history of a pre-existing hernia. Operative repair can be via a high, modified high or low approach. The Lichtenstein repair is for inguinal hernias.

4.44 A. True
  B. True
  C. True
  D. True
  E. True

All of these are different ways of repairing inguinal hernias and the candidate must consult appropriate texts for the full description.

4.45 A. True
  B. True
  C. False
  D. False
  E. False

Mortality of elective hernia repair according to age is : < 60 – 0.1%; 60–69 – 0.2%; 70–79 – 1.6%; >80 – 3.3%. The mortality of strangulated hernia repair is around 13%. Ten per cent of patients with strangulation give no previous history of a hernia. Richter's hernia is a partial enterocele which undergoes strangulation and obstruction. Maydl's hernia has a W-loop strangulation with the strangulated bowel within the abdominal cavity. Littre's hernia is a strangulated Meckel's diverticulum, and this can cause a small bowel fistula. Inguinal hernias can be repaired as day cases under general anaesthesia. The use of non-absorbable mesh is advised. Patients should avoid sports for at least six weeks after repair.

4.46 A. True
  B. True
  C. False
  D. True
  E. True

The femoral canal lies medial to the femoral vein, has the inguinal ligament as its anterior border, the lacunar ligament as its medial border, the pectineal ligament as its posterior border and contains the lymph node of Cloquet.

4.47 A. True
   B. True
   C. False
   D. True
   E. False

Almost 100 000 hernia operations are performed annually in the UK. The hernial contents form part of the sac wall in a sliding hernia. The cremasteric muscle does not play any part in inguinal hernia repair. Persistent groin pain may be a result of ilioinguinal nerve entrapment in the repair scar.

4.48 A. False
   B. True
   C. False
   D. False
   E. False

A truly strangulated inguinal hernia causing intestinal obstruction needs to be surgically repaired as an emergency. It is however not an indication for a full laparotomy. Bowel resection renders the operation 'dirty' and is thus a contraindication to the use of mesh. The patient need not be managed on i.v. fluids and NG tube.

4.49 A. True
   B. True
   C. True
   D. True
   E. True

Non-specific acute abdominal pain can be caused by all of the following: irritable bowel syndrome, viral infections, gastroenteritis, nerve root pain and psychosomatic pain.

4.50 A. True
   B. False
   C. True
   D. False
   E. False

Although blood tests are often useful as a baseline, their influence on the diagnosis of acute abdominal pain remains unclear, with the exception of serum amylase for acute pancreatitis. Serial white-cell counts are useful as compared with a single measurement. Liver function tests are extremely useful in confirming or refuting acute biliary disease but not the presence or absence of gallstones. Metabolic acidosis is often a late change in intestinal ischaemia.

4.51 A. True
   B. False
   C. False
   D. False
   E. False

Erect CXR is the most appropriate investigation in suspected free intraperitoneal gas. Lateral decubitus film can be used if erect CXR cannot be taken (for example, because of the patient's condition). Radiologists consider that the supine abdominal film is sufficient to diagnose obstruction. Erect CXR shows no free gas in approximately 30–50% of cases with perforated viscus. This leaves three management options: (1) reconsider the diagnosis; (2) proceed to laparotomy; and (3) water-soluble contrast study if there are reasonable grounds for not proceeding with laparotomy. Emergency ultrasound of the abdomen does not reliably image the pancreas. Urine microscopy is necessary especially if the diagnosis is doubtful.

4.52 A. True
   B. True
   C. False
   D. False
   E. True

Improved capillary return, slowing of tachycardia and normalization of blood pressure and pulse pressure are signs of return of organ perfusion and indicate fluid resuscitation. Bladder catheterization allows accurate measurement of urine output, and satisfactory diuresis suggests adequate fluid replacement. In severe shock, mental function may be impaired and improved consciousness is a favourable sign.

4.53 A. False
   B. True
   C. False
   D. True
   E. True

Significant amounts of fluid and electrolyte may be sequestered with an inflamed peritoneal cavity or obstructed bowel. In the presence of sepsis, expansion of the interstitial space may be associated with a relative intravascular hypovolaemia. In the previously healthy adult, up to 1500 ml of fluid may be lost before physical signs are obvious. Significant acute fluid loss (more than 15% of circulating volume) will be recognized by the classical signs of hypovolaemic shock. Systolic hypotension may not be manifest until more than 30% of circulating volume has been lost. Gastrointestinal fluid losses are best replaced with crystalloid fluids. When there is relative hypovolaemia secondary to sepsis, colloid replacement with plasma or a synthetic substitute can be considered. If there is concomitant anaemia, blood is preferable.

Electrolyte losses as a result of acute gastrointestinal disease may be considerable. Diarrhoea and loss of colonic mucus may cause hypokalaemia. Hyponatraemia may be caused by profuse vomiting or sepsis. Correction of hyponatraemia should not delay appropriate surgical intervention.

4.54 A. False
   B. True
   C. True
   D. False
   E. True

Peutz–Jeghers syndrome is inherited as autosomal dominant. It often presents with anaemia in childhood and is characterized by circumoral mucocutaneous pigmented lesions. The polyps are hamartomatous. Malignant change does occur in 2–3% of polyps.

4.55 A. False
   B. True
   C. False
   D. True
   E. True

H. pylori is Gram negative. Duodenal ulceration is more common than oesophageal. Zollinger–Ellison syndrome is associated with gastrin hypersecretion. PPIs will heal 95% of duodenal ulcers in six weeks. Triple therapy (omeprazole, metronidazole and ampicillin) can eradicate *H. pylori*.

4.56 A. True
   B. False
   C. True
   D. False
   E. True

Pancreatic carcinoma can present with pain, weight loss and obstructive jaundice. Eighty per cent are in the head of the gland. Pancreatic cancers are ductal adenocarcinomas in 90% of cases. They can be detected by ultrasound scan, CT scans or other imaging modality. Most cases are found late, and are therefore unsuitable for curative surgery.

4.57 A. True
   B. True
   C. True
   D. True
   E. True

Acute appendicitis is commonest in childhood. Mortality increases with age and is greatest in the elderly. The commonest lie of the appendix is in a retrocaecal position. Faecoliths may be present in resected specimens. Appendicitis is a possible diagnosis in the absence of pyrexia.

4.58 A. True
   B. False
   C. False
   D. False
   E. True

Gallbladder stones are mostly composed of cholesterol. Pigment stones are a result of increased unconjugated bilirubin. Only 10% are radio-opaque. They are a risk factor for the development of gallbladder carcinoma. When impacted in Hartmann's pouch they can cause mucocele of the gallbladder.

4.59 A. True
   B. True
   C. True
   D. True
   E. False

Common bile duct calculi are found in over 10% of patients undergoing cholecystectomy. They can present with Charcot's Triad – fever, rigors jaundice. They are suggested by a bile duct diameter > 8 mm on ultrasound, and are best treated by ERCP, sphincterotomy and balloon clearance. The T-tube can safely be removed after ten days.

4.60 A. False
  B. True
  C. True
  D. False
  E. True

Ulcerative colitis is confined to the mucosa. It always involves the rectum and extends proximally along the colon, and may even affect the terminal ileal (backwash ileitis). Crohn's disease causes fistulae in 10% of cases, but not ulcerative colitis. UC spares the serosa of the colon.

4.61 A. False
  B. False
  C. True
  D. True
  E. False

Patients with total colitis may require surgery after ten years to prevent malignant transformation. Panproctocolectomy and pouch formation is inappropriate as an emergency operation, and the surgery of choice should be total colectomy with colostomy formation and oversewing of the rectal stump. Pouches can be fashioned as 'S', 'J' or 'W' loops. Patients with a successful pouch are continent for stools. With a pouch the mean stool frequency is about up to six times per day.

4.62 A. False
  B. False
  C. True
  D. True
  E. True

Anal fissures commonly occur in the posterior midline of the anal canal. They may heal with the use of a bulking agent, or be treated with sphincterotomy which is safer than Lord's procedure. Sphincterotomy could lead to incontinence. Recurrence does not necessarily suggest Crohn's disease.

4.63 **A.** False
   B. False
   C. True
   D. False
   E. True

Familial adenomatous polyposis (FAP) is an autosomal dominant condition and is characterized by polyp formation in late adolescence. It is associated with osteomas and epidermoid cysts in Gardner syndrome. It is caused by a mutation on chromosome 5. It can be screened for by rigid or flexible sigmoidoscopy, or colonoscopy.

4.64 **A.** False
   B. False
   C. False
   D. True
   E. False

The rectum is the commonest site of colorectal tumours. It is predisposed by dysplastic polyps, not metaplastic polyps. Local recurrence is decreased by total mesorectal excision. When in the upper third of the rectum, it is most appropriately managed by an anterior resection. Chemotherapy is not of proven benefit in Dukes' A tumours.

4.65 **A.** False
   B. False
   C. True
   D. False
   E. False

Oesophageal cancer cannot be eradicated by large-scale screening programmes. It does not arise commonly in Barrett's oesophagus. Its incidence is related to environmental factors. It can be curable surgically. Palliation with a metallic stent is usually successful.

4.66 A. True
   B. True
   C. True
   D. False

Failure of endoscopic control of active bleeding and recurrent bleeding after endoscopic control are strong indications for surgery. In the over-60 age group and in those who have received transfusion of more than four units of blood, surgery has been shown in trials to be the safest management with better outcome. The size of the ulcer on its own is immaterial.

4.67 A. False
   B. False
   C. False
   D. True
   E. False

For many years the standard treatment was truncal vagotomy and drainage, and when a gastrectomy was necessary, a vagotomy was often added. The rationale behind this approach was to provide definitive therapy and thereby minimize the risk of life-threatening recurrence. Over the past ten years the medical treatment of peptic ulcer has improved. Although ineffective in stopping bleeding, H2 receptor antagonists or the proton pump inhibitors are best and most effective in securing ulcer healing. The pathogenic role of *Helicobacter* is now firmly established and successful eradication therapy reduces the risk of recurrent ulcer to very acceptable levels; no surgical procedure is therefore necessary. Pylorus-preserving duodenectomy is not a recognized surgical procedure.

4.68 A. False
   B. True
   C. True
   D. False
   E. True

The causes of acute life-threatening colonic bleeding include angiodysplasia, diverticulosis and ulcerative colitis.

4.69 A. True
B. True
C. False
D. True
E. False

In one study angiodysplasias were an incidental finding in 6% of all colonoscopies and up to 20% of the elderly.

In 80% of patients angiodysplasia affects the terminal ileum, caecum, ascending colon or hepatic inflexure, while 20% are present in the descending colon and sigmoid. Associations with coagulopathy and cardiac valvular disease are frequently quoted and were noted in 28% and 25% respectively of the cases in one study. Angiodysplasia presents in a variety of ways ranging from unexplained iron deficiency anaemia to acute colonic haemorrhage. Dilated tortuous vessels and distinct 'cherry red' areas are features of angiodysplasia on colonoscopy. In the acute setting and without optimum bowel preparation the relatively subtle appearances are easily missed and the diagnosis is often dependent on arteriography.

4.70 A. True
B. True
C. True
D. True
E. False

The causes of small bowel obstruction include Crohn's disease strictures, adhesions from previous abdominal surgery, diaphragmatic hernias and carcinoma of the caecum.

4.71 A. True
  B. False
  C. False
  D. True
  E. False

The typical clinical presentation of small bowel obstruction is central abdominal colicky pain, vomiting – which is often bile stained – abdominal distension and a reduction or absence of flatus. Vomiting may be less of a feature and a greater degree of abdominal distension observed if the blockage is in the distal ileum. Bowel sounds increase. Localized peritonitic pain and tenderness may develop. The presence of surgical scars is important as is any history of previous intra-abdominal pathology.

4.72 A. True
  B. False
  C. False
  D. False
  E. True

The first step is resuscitation of the patient with intravenous fluids and administration of supplemental oxygen. Urinary catheterization and central venous pressure management, particularly in elderly patients or those with co-existing morbidity, is essential. Adequate fluid replacement must be given rapidly if surgical intervention is planned. Decompression of the stomach with a nasogastric tube will reduce vomiting in most patients, decompress the bowel and reduce the risk of airway contamination by aspiration. Fluid lost via the nasogastric tube should be replaced with additional intravenous crystalloids and potassium. Analgesia should be given early and in adequate doses. The analgesia requirement needs to be reviewed regularly in the early stages of management and opiates are generally required, intravenously if necessary (for instance in the hypovolaemic patient). These will not mask signs of localized or generalized peritonitis and there is no justification for withholding adequate analgesia while waiting for further clinical assessment.

4.73 A. False
     B. True
     C. False
     D. True
     E. False

Delayed presentation or surgery commonly results in gangrene of the affected bowel. Surgery is mandatory; manipulating the hernia risks reducing gangrenous bowel or non-resolution of the obstruction. The hernia is repaired in the usual way including the use of mesh despite the slight increase in risk of complications which are minimized by treatment with antibiotics.

4.74 A. True
     B. False
     C. False
     D. False
     E. False

Peak incidence in the UK is towards 30 years of age. Acute appendicitis is caused by luminal blockage – for example by faecoliths – and not direct infection. Appendicular masses are only managed conservatively in stable, well patients when it is assumed that the risk of diffuse peritonitis has passed. If the patient deteriorates then it is likely that assumption is false and surgery is necessary. Ultrasound scanning is by no means accurate in diagnosing acute appendicitis, however recent studies favour focal CT scanning where the appendicular wall thickness appears to be an accurate indicator of appendicitis.

4.75 A. False
     B. True
     C. False
     D. True
     E. False

The incidence of perforated peptic ulcer is falling. It can be caused by steroid therapy. Conservative management can be tried if the contrast study demonstrates no leak. The ulcers can be treated laparoscopically. Air under the diaphragm is present in only around 65–70% of cases.

4.76 A. True
   B. False
   C. False
   D. False
   E. False

Algorithm of the management of massive rectal bleeding (non-haemorroidal) of unknown site:

Stable patient → colonoscopy → Angiography +/– embolization → labelled red-cell scan

$$\downarrow \qquad\qquad\qquad \downarrow$$

Unstable patient → gastroscopy → laparotomy +/– intraoperative endoscopy.

4.77 A. True
   B. True
   C. True
   D. True
   E. True

The presenting features of sepsis and systemic inflammatory response syndrome (SIRS) include haemorrhage and bruising, lactic acidosis, acute respiratory distress syndrome, and both hyper- and hypothermia.

4.78 A. True
    B. False
    C. False
    D. False
    E. True

Cardiovascular failure = one or more of the following:
1. Mean arterial pressure less than 49 mmHg.
2. Ventricular tachycardia/fibrillation.
3. Serum pH less than 7.24 (perfusion related).
4. Acute complete heart block
5. Use of vasoactive drugs to support arterial pressure.

Respiratory failure = one or more of the following:
1. Respiratory rate greater than 49 min.
2. P_aCO_2 greater than 50 mmHg in the absence of opiate drugs or metabolic alkalosis.
3. Dependence on mechanical ventilation for more than 12 h.

Renal failure = one or more of the following:
1. Oliguria (less than 0.5 ml/kg/h urine output) with elevated creatinine despite adequate fluids.
2. Serum urea greater than 35 mmol.
3. Serum creatinine greater than 300 mmol.

Haematological failure = one or more of the following:
1. WBC less than 1000 mm.
2. Platelets less than 20 000 mm.
3. Haematocrit less than 20% in the absence of bleeding.

Neurological failure = either:
1. Best Glasgow Coma Scale less than 8.
2. Neuropathy, myopathy or cord lesion limiting respirator mobility.

4.79 A. True
    B. True
    C. True
    D. True
    E. True

The factors contributing to the development of MODS include uncontrolled sepsis, massive fluid/volume resuscitation, hypovolaemic shock, specific organ disease and crush injuries.

4.80 A. True
  B. True
  C. False
  D. False
  E. True

Some patients are more susceptible to septic complications than others. Systemic inflammatory response syndrome (SIRS) is thought to be a result of inadequate or overwhelmed local host defence mechanisms. SIRS does not result only from infections and does not usually respond to intravenous antibiotic therapy. When caused by bacteria, sepsis and SIRS are synonymous.

4.81 1. B
  2. E

4.82 1. A
  2. F
  3. D

In vascular surgery the commonest infecting organisms are *Staphylococcus aureus* and coagulase negative Staphylococcus. They are most simply prevented by the use of a single dose of augmentin. Prostatic biopsy may be complicated by a Gram-negative bacteraemia. The prophylaxis most commonly used is either a single injection of gentamicin or ciprofloxacin.

Colonic surgery requires broad-spectrum antibiotics and anaerobic cover. A combination of antibiotics is usually employed, cefuroxime and metronidazole or ciprofloxacin and metronidazole.

4.83 1. D
     2. C

Arterial anastomoses require non-absorbable sutures of sufficient strength that pull through tissues easily. An aortic anastomosis requires the strength of a 2/0 suture. Intestinal anastomoses utilize absorbable sutures: 2/0 PDS would be the most appropriate of the sutures listed for a gastrojejunostomy. No. 1 loop nylon is generally used for mass closure of the abdomen.

Urinary system and renal transplantation

URINARY SYSTEM

5.1 **A.** False
    B. True
    C. True
    D. False
    E. True

The diagnosis of bladder cancer is made on cystoscopy, biopsy or resection of the tumour with histology. CT scans have a role in the staging of bladder cancer, that is, the local extent of the tumour and the presence of pelvic and para-aortic lymphadenopathy. Haematuria is present in 85–90% of patients. It can be micro- or macroscopic, and is quite often intermittent. Cigarette smokers have up to a fourfold higher incidence of transitional cell carcinoma of the bladder than non-smokers. The risk correlates with the number of cigarettes consumed, the duration of smoking and the depth of inhalation. Interestingly, the reduction of risk down to baseline following cessation takes at least 20 years, which is far longer than the reduction of risk for cardiovascular and pulmonary disease. Transitional cell carcinoma of the bladder does not usually metastasize to renal parenchyma. However, the urothelium of the ureter and renal pelvis is at a slightly increased risk of developing transitional cell carcinoma. The most important prognostic factors are tumour grade, stage and presence of carcinoma in situ. Other important factors include tumour size (>10 g), multi-focality and frequency of recurrence.

5.2 **A.** True
B. True
C. True
D. False
E. True

A three-way urethral catheter should be inserted to wash out the blood clots to prevent clot retention. Once the blood clots are washed out, the haematuria will very often settle, especially after transurethral resection of the prostate. Microscopy, culture and sensitivity of the urine are essential investigations to confirm haematuria and to exclude urinary tract infection. Patients with macroscopic haematuria should have their upper tract imaged by an intravenous urogram (IVU) and/or ultrasound. While a large bladder tumour will be detected on IVU or US, small ones may be missed and therefore a cystoscopy should also be performed. Radio-nuclide renogram does not have a role in the initial investigation of haematuria. A good quality IVU will pick up most transitional cell carcinomas of the renal pelvis and ureter. If the suspicion of renal cell carcinoma is high, an ultrasound of the kidneys should also be performed.

5.3 **A.** False
B. True
C. False
D. False
E. True

The ureter has three narrowings: (1) at the pelvi-ureteric junction; (2) at the point where it crosses the iliac vessels; and (3) at the vesico-ureteric junction, where it is narrowest. Ureteric calculi are often impacted at these locations. The ureter is lined by a transitional cell epithelium, identical and contiguous with that of the urinary bladder and the renal pelvis. The majority of transitional cell carcinomas of the urothelium involve the urinary bladder (90%). Nine per cent involve the renal pelvis and only 1% involve the ureter. The ureter is closely related to the uterine cervix and is crossed anteriorly by the uterine artery; it is therefore at risk during hysterectomy. Pathology of the fallopian tubes or ovaries may involve the ureter at the pelvic brim level. The ureter receives sympathetic input from T10 and L2. Its parasympathetic supply comes from S2–4. However, normal ureteric peristalsis does not require autonomic input. It originates and is propagated from intrinsic smooth muscle pacemaker sites in the minor calyces of the collecting system.

5.4 **A.** False
 B. True
 C. False
 D. True
 E. False

An obstructed kidney with superimposed infection is a urological emergency. The immediate objective is to relieve the obstruction safely and efficiently, either via a percutaneous nephrostomy or antegrade ureteric stent under antibiotic cover, with close monitoring of the patient, watching for septicaemia. Neither ESWL nor ureteroscopy can guarantee complete and immediate clearance of the ureteric stone to decompress the kidney. It is essential to know what organism is growing in the urine because antibiotic is almost always required in these patients, who are at high risk of septicaemia. The indication to catheterize in this case is to monitor urine output in a patient who is in septic shock. Elderly patients with pre-existing impaired cardiorespiratory function would require further monitoring, for example by central venous pressure line. Such patients are usually septicaemic and blood culture should always be taken.

5.5 **A.** True
    B. False
    C. False
    D. False
    E. True

Bladder calculi present predominantly in men over 50 and are associated with bladder outflow obstruction. The diagnosis and management of bladder calculus should encompass factors that cause bladder outflow obstruction, for example prostatic enlargement, urethral stricture, bladder diverticulum and neurogenic bladder. Hyperoxaluria is not a common cause of bladder calculi which are usually composed of uric acid (in non-infected urine) or struvite (in infected urine). The presence of oxalate in a bladder calculus is suggestive of a renal origin. The best treatment of bladder calculi is their removal plus the elimination of the predisposing causes. Instillation of Suby's G solution does have a role in the reduction of recurrence in bladder calculi in patients with a long-term catheter in situ. Uric acid bladder calculi can be present in up to 50% of cases. Uric acid stones are radiolucent. In addition, small bladder calculi may not show up on plain KUB. Cystoscopy is therefore also required.

5.6 **A.** True
    B. True
    C. False
    D. True
    E. False

Bladder outflow obstruction can lead to detrusor instability or decreased compliance and frequency and urgency will result. Hyperglycosuria in uncontrolled diabetics can cause lower urinary tract symptoms. Their urinary frequency can also be exacerbated by their polyuria and diabetic neuropathy. Patients should have further investigations to elucidate the cause before an anticholinergic is used. Caffeine, for example in tea and coffee, cigarettes and alcohol are bladder stimulants in some patients. If bladder outflow obstruction secondary to prostatic hyperplasia is the cause, transurethral resection of the prostate is likely to improve these symptoms.

5.7 **A.** False
B. True
C. False
D. False
E. False

Evidence from prospective trials (the American Urological Association BPH Treatment Outcome Study) suggests that there is no significant correlation between the severity of symptoms and prostate size. There are no absolute indications for open prostatectomy in benign prostate gland. However, it is accepted practice to limit transurethral resection time to 1 h and therefore most urologists will elect to remove a 150 g benign prostate via the open retropubic route. There are only a few absolute contraindications to urethral catheterization, such as the presence of blood at the urethral meatus after suspected pelvic fracture and urethral rupture. There is no good evidence at present to suggest that benign prostatic hyperplasia is a risk factor for the subsequent development of adenocarcinoma of the prostate. LHRH analogues are used in the treatment of adenocarcinoma of the prostate and not benign prostatic hyperplasia. 5-alpha reductase inhibitor (finasteride) is one of the best medical treatments for benign prostatic hyperplasia.

5.8 **A.** False
    B. True
    C. False
    D. False
    E. True

The indication for radical prostatectomy is a localized adenocarcinoma of the prostate in a surgically fit patient with a reasonable life expectancy of more than ten years. It is not beneficial to patients with metastasis. Symptomatic metastatic carcinoma of the prostate should be treated by hormonal manipulation, that is, surgical or medical castration, luteinizing hormone releasing hormone analogue, or an antiandrogen licensed for monotherapy such as cyproterone acetate. The probability of developing prostate cancer is less than 1 in 10 000 in men aged under 40, 1 in 103 for men between 40 and 59 and 1 in 8 for men between 60 and 79. Metastatic carcinoma of the prostate causing spinal cord compression is a neurological emergency and should be referred immediately for neurosurgical cord decompression or radiotherapy. Once paralysis is established, recovery of motor function is poor. There is a place for low-dose stilboestrol as second-line hormonal treatment of metastatic cancer of the prostate. Antiandrogen therapy such as cyproterone acetate or flutamide is used to prevent 'tumour flare' caused by the initial surge of serum testosterone induced by luteinizing hormone releasing hormone analogue. Orchidectomy does not induce this transient rise of testosterone and therefore 'tumour flare' does not happen.

5.9 **A.** False
    B. False
    C. False
    D. False
    E. True

Serum PSA elevation can occur after any procedure or process that disrupts the normal architecture, for example prostatic cancer, benign prostatic hyperplasia and prostatitis, as well as manipulation such as prostatic massage, biopsy and digital rectal examination. However, the elevation after a digital rectal examination appears to be within the error of the assay and rarely causes a false-positive result. Non-prostatic sources of PSA include amniotic fluid, ovarian endothelium and cancer of colon, lung, pancreas, kidney or adrenal gland, and breast cancer in women. PSA production by malignant prostate cells is variable and depends on the degree of differentiation, with poorly differentiated cancer producing less PSA. Twenty-five per cent of men with prostate cancer have PSA levels less than 4.0 ng/ml, the level used as the upper limit of normal in most studies using the Hybritech Tandem assay. PSA is a serine protease produced by the prostatic epithelium and periurethral gland in the male. It is secreted in high concentration in the semen and is involved in the liquefaction of the semen coagulum.

5.10 **A.** False
    B. False
    C. False
    D. True
    E. False

BPH arises in the transition zone of the prostate which is just outside the urethra at the verumontanum, and does not occur in the whole gland. Seventy per cent of prostate cancers arise in the peripheral zone of the prostate. The first change of BPH occurs at about 35 years of age and consists of microscopic stromal nodules around the periurethral glands. Glandular hyperplasia occurs around these nodules, which may be predominantly glandular, or stromal, or of mixed composition. Studies have estimated that in BPH, PSA elevation is proportional to the size of the transition zone. 1 g of BPH is thought to elevate PSA by 0.3 ng/dl. Other important causes of elevated PSA are prostate cancer and prostatitis.

5.11 A. False
  B. True
  C. False
  D. True
  E. True

Testicular torsion can be intra- or extravaginal. Extravaginal occurs almost exclusively in neonates or in utero. Infants usually present with a painless scrotal swelling. Intravaginal torsion occurs at all ages but most commonly in adolescents. It is associated with a high insertion of the tunica vaginalis on the cord, which allows the testicle to twist.

The torted testicle usually has a high and transverse lie. Elevation of the testicle usually relieves the pain of epididymitis but not the pain of torsion. Surgical exploration remains the best diagnostic test for a possible testicular torsion. The testicle usually twists medially and can rotate 720°. With suitable analgesia manual detorsion can be attempted by lateral rotation of the testicle for two full twists (720°). Torsion can permanently affect spermatogenesis after 4–6 h. Leydig cell function is more resistant to hypoxia. After 24 h of torsion the testicle will not be salvageable.

5.12 A. True
  B. False
  C. True
  D. False
  E. True

Any aetiology causing spinal cord compression can cause acute urinary retention and neurological causes should be excluded in all these patients. It is also common in postoperative patients who have had epidural anaesthesia, and can also be caused by benign prostatic hyperplasia, bladder-neck contractions and urethral strictures. Drugs may also affect bladder function and in patients with a degree of outflow obstruction can push the patient into retention. These include anticholinergics, drugs with some anticholinergic effects and antihistamines.

5.13 A. False
   B. True
   C. True
   D. False
   E. False

Lower urinary tract symptoms can be assessed by a symptom score, that is, the International Prostate Symptom Score. A high score does not however necessarily correlate with bladder outflow obstruction. If the flow rate is < 10 ml/s there is an 82% chance that the patient is obstructed. Large post-void residuals correlate better with detrusor failure rather than bladder outflow obstruction. Sphincter dyssynergia, seen in spinal cord injuries, can cause bladder outflow obstruction as the sphincter contracts instead of relaxing when the bladder contracts. Urethral but not ureteric strictures can cause bladder outflow obstruction.

5.14 A. True
   B. True
   C. True
   D. False
   E. False

Blunt renal injuries can be divided into 5 grades from grade 1, which is a minor contusion, to grade 5, which is a shattered kidney or an avulsed pedicle. Adults with blunt trauma and microscopic haematuria but no shock have a very low incidence of major renal trauma and do not need any further radiological imaging of the kidneys. Gross haematuria increases the rate of major renal trauma to 12.5%. All blunt renal trauma patients with gross haematuria or microscopic haematuria who are shocked need renal imaging with IVU, CT or angiography if pedicle injury is suspected. Renal trauma can still occur in the absence of haematuria. Four absolute indications for exploration are an expanding haematoma, pulsatile haematoma, life-threatening haemodynamic instability and known grade 5 renal injury. Most minor injuries can be managed conservatively.

5.15 A. True
   B. True
   C. False
   D. False
   E. True

Vesico-ureteric reflux predisposes infection and the infection causes reflux nephropathy. The normal mechanism for preventing reflux is the oblique passage of the ureter through the bladder wall which creates a valve-like mechanism. The ratio between the length of the ureteric tunnel and the diameter of the ureter is important and should usually exceed 4:1. Lateral placement of the ureteric orifices as found in duplex systems (lower moiety) causes a shorter, more direct passage through the bladder wall and predisposes to reflux. In infants and children the ureter tends to have a more direct passage and reflux is common. Most children with mild to moderate reflux can be managed conservatively as the reflux will tend to improve with age.

5.16 1. A
   2. B
   3. C

Patient 1 has recurrence of his outflow obstruction, for example by bladder-neck stenosis and urethral stricture, both of which are late complications of TURP. There is a higher incidence of bladder-neck stenosis after transurethral resection of a small prostate and, in such cases, bladder-neck incision may be more appropriate.

   Patient 2 is a classical presentation of advanced metastatic carcinoma of the prostate. His back pain is caused by bony metastasis or ureteric obstruction as a result of local involvement of the prostate cancer at the distal ureter. The treatment in such cases would involve hormonal manipulation. A large proportion of patients will show good response initially but most will eventually relapse after a variable period of time.

   Patient 3 is a typical presentation of obstructive uropathy as a result of prostatic enlargement of a longstanding nature as shown by the dilated upper tract, thinning of renal cortex and anaemia. This situation is one of the few absolute indications for a prostatectomy.

5.17 **1.** C
2. D
3. E
4. F
5. C

Patient 1 is most likely to have a transitional cell carcinoma of the bladder at the left ureteric orifice causing obstruction to the left kidney. If the filling defect was in the ureter, differential diagnoses would include both A and B.

Patient 2 has renal angiolyomyoma associated with tuberous sclerosis (the sign of adenoma sebaceum on her face). A characteristic feature on the CT scan is a mass – predominantly of fat. The first-line definitive treatment in cases of severe bleeding is selective embolization, aiming to preserve renal function. If this fails and significant bleeding persists, partial nephrectomy is required.

Patient 3 has renal cell carcinoma with tumour thrombus in the inferior vena cava causing obstruction to the venous drainage of his lower limbs. His fever, fatigue and weight loss are part of the syndrome of reversible hepatic dysfunction associated with renal cell carcinoma.

Patient 4 is a classical presentation of retroperitoneal fibrosis. It is important to exclude malignancy (including Hodgkin's lymphoma, breast and colonic cancer). Methysergide has been implicated. Other causes include inflammatory aortic aneurysm and inflammatory bowel disease. Treatment is usually surgical (ureterolysis) which include biopsy of the fibrous plaque to exclude malignancy, although steroids have been used when the disease is mild and bilateral ureteric stenting has its place in patients not fit for major surgery.

With patient 5, this is a common presentation of bladder cancer. The filling defect can also be caused by a large blood clot but in either case, he would require a rigid cystoscopy, bladder washout and resection of the bladder tumour if one is present.

5.18 1. B
    2. D

TUR syndrome, seen in patient 1, occurs in about 2% of patients in some series. It is caused by dilutional hyponatraemia. Affected patients usually become symptomatic when their serum sodium is less than 125 mmol/l. The risk of developing TUR syndrome is increased by a large gland and prolonged (> 90 min) resection time. The use of warm irrigation fluid helps to reduce the risk. In addition, should there be a large prostatic capsular perforation with opening of the venous sinus, haemostasis should be obtained promptly and the resection terminated. Treatment of TUR syndrome consists of judicious administration of hypertonic saline and frusemide.

    A cause of lower abdominal pain after transurethral surgery, seen in patient 2, is fluid extravasation as a result of bladder perforation during resection of bladder tumour. It is best to exercise extra care when resecting or performing biopsy at the vault of the bladder where it is thin, especially in women.

5.19 1. D
    2. E

There are several testicular appendages, the most common being the appendix testi and the appendix of the epididymis. They can both undergo torsion and mimic testicular torsion. If seen early, a small nodule can be seen on the superior pole of the testicle. This appears as a black or blue dot through the scrotal skin (The Blue/Black Dot Sign).

    When examining a scrotal lump several questions should always be answered as this will help in diagnosing the correct condition. In this case the swelling was not confined to the scrotum making the diagnosis of a hernia or communicating hydrocele most likely. The testicle was felt as a separate structure and the swelling did not transilluminate so it was not a hydrocele.

5.20 1. E
2. A
3. I

Seminomas of the testicle are homogeneous masses whilst teratomas are likely to be heterogeneous. On section the seminoma has the appearance of a cut potato. Whilst testicular tumours cause elevation of tumour markers in about 70% of cases, pure seminomas do not produce alpha fetoprotein. In the event of histology showing a seminoma, if the alpha fetoprotein is elevated then the pathologist should re-examine the sample, as there will be a teratomatous element within it.

Undescended testicle predisposes to testicular tumours and increases the risk eightfold. The risk is not only in the undescended testicle but also in the normally descended one (in unilateral maldescent). Undescended testicles predispose to seminomas.

As the testicle is non-tender on examination it is not likely to be torsion of the testicle or epididymitis. The urine had blood but no traces of leucocytes or nitrates. This would favour a ureteric stone as the cause of the pain but this should be confirmed by intravenous urogram.

RENAL TRANSPLANTATION

5.21 A. False
    B. False
    C. False
    D. True
    E. False

HIV positivity, if confirmed by Western blotting, remains an absolute contraindication to organ transplantation. Oxalosis recurs in the transplant kidney and it remains a relative contraindication but simultaneous liver and kidney transplantation will give prolonged survival. Focal sclerosis is also known to recur in renal transplant but it does not remain an absolute contraindication. Hepatitis C patients can be transplanted provided liver function is satisfactory. Chronic pyelonephritis is acceptable provided its cause is treated.

5.22 A. True
    B. False
    C. True
    D. False
    E. False

Patients with CRF often need to remain on dialysis for many years. Both peritoneal dialysis and haemodialysis are acceptable though haemodialysis is preferred. In anticipation of end-stage renal failure, either a PD catheter or AV fistula must be sited. Bilateral nephrectomy should only be considered if there is uncontrolled hypertension, proteinuria or infection. Renal biopsy and cystoscopy are not always indicated.

5.23 A. False
    B. False
    C. True
    D. False

Long-term studies have shown no decrease in survival or renal dysfunction in living kidney donors who are prepared adequately and no advantage is gained from using an older or younger donor, provided renal function in the particular individual is satisfactory. Since the histocompatibility is inherited in a Mendelian fashion, 25% of siblings will be a perfect match resulting in 95–98% long-term graft survival.

5.24 A. True
    B. True
    C. False
    D. False
    E. False

ABO incompatibility and a current positive T-cell crossmatch are absolute contraindications to cadaveric renal transplant. Historic positive crossmatches with a current T-cell crossmatch, while important, do not contraindicate a transplant. Cold ischaemia time, while accounting for delayed function, does not matter. Multiple arteries can increase the technical difficulty of the transplant operation, but do not constitute an absolute contraindication.

5.25 A. True
    B. True
    C. False
    D. True
    E. True

The diagnosis of brain death is made on the basis of irrefutable clinical documentation of irreversible absence of cerebral and brainstem function. While a flat EEG can support the diagnosis, it is not mandatory. Other causes of cerebral dysfunction such as hypothermia, endocrine disturbance and drug overdose must also be excluded.

5.26 A. False
    B. True
    C. False
    D. False
    E. False

The most common cause of initial non-function of a cadaveric graft is acute tubular necrosis, and this is related to prolonged warm or cold ischaemia times. However the sudden cessation of urine output in a previously functioning transplant kidney, in the absence of a catheter block, is almost always the result of an arterial or venous thrombosis. While ultrasound and Doppler assessment are useful if available, urgent exploration provides the quickest and best chance of salvaging kidney function. Diuresis, antibiotics and antirejection treatment are not indicated in this situation.

5.27 A. True
  B. False
  C. False
  D. True
  E. False

The use of the internal iliac artery has been abandoned as bilateral internal iliac ligation can result in erectile impotence in young men. It is indeed preferable to assess the patency and bloodflow in the pelvic blood vessels prior to transplantation if there is a possibility of underlying vascular disease, but is not always mandatory. The vascular anastomoses are usually carried out to the iliac blood vessels in an adult.

5.28 A. True
  B. False
  C. False
  D. True
  E. False

Viral infections and an increased potential for malignancy remain a threat to all transplant patients. There is no evidence that immunosuppression is teratogenic: in fact many successful and normal pregnancies have been reported following transplantation. There is certainly no requirement to isolate or prevent patients from returning to work.

5.29 A. False
  B. False
  C. True
  D. False
  E. False

Immunosuppression does not pose a threat to a pregnancy. Patients should neither stop nor increase their immunosuppression. All patients should monitor BP and other parameters of renal function.

5.30 A. False
   B. False
   C. False
   D. True
   E. True

Regulation of blood pressure is crucial in post-transplant management. A diagnosis of a critical renal artery stenosis calls for urgent treatment with balloon angioplasty, failing which surgical exploration is mandatory.

5.31 A. True
   B. False
   C. True
   D. True
   E. False

Anti-HLA antibodies develop in response to exposure to foreign antigens either from earlier blood transfusions, pregnancy or prior transplants. The titre and specificity of the antibodies are significant factors in acute rejection.

5.32 A. True
   B. False
   C. False
   D. False
   E. False

Any form of vascular access has thrombosis or stenosis as a potential complication. AV fistulae have the best patency rates and all other forms of artificial device suffer a higher failure rate.

5.33 A. True
   B. True
   C. True
   D. True
   E. True

5.34 A. True
   B. True
   C. True
   D. True

The initial management will consist of continued PD exchanges with added antibiotics. If this does not resolve the problem laparotomy and removal of the infected PD catheter, with conversion to haemodialysis, will be necessary.

5.35 A. False
   B. True
   C. True
   D. False
   E. False

Cyclosporin toxicity is a possibility, though assuming that the levels have been correctly monitored the most likely cause is acute rejection. Renal vein thrombosis would present as an acute renal shutdown. Renal artery stenosis and viral infections such as CMV are more likely to be delayed complications.

5.36 A. True
   B. False
   C. True
   D. True
   E. False

Ultrasonography provides the best help in assessing obstruction or swelling of the kidney. Renography will provide evidence of renal perfusion. Reduction of cyclosporin without assessment of drug levels is unsafe. A transplant biopsy is the best method of assessing any pathological process in the kidney.

5.37 A. False
   B. True
   C. False
   D. True
   E. True

PTLD is usually a B-cell non-Hodgkin's lymphoma (96%) and has a mortality rate 50 times higher than for lymphomas in the general population. PTLD may respond to withdrawal of immunosuppression or antiviral agents.

5.38 A. False
  B. False
  C. False
  E. True
  F. False

Prophylactic antibiotics and the reduction of immunosuppression have only a minimal role in transplantation. While isolation of patients was practised many years ago, it is not now considered necessary. Treatment of a focus of infection prior to transplant is essential to avoid post-transplant problems of overwhelming sepsis following immunosuppression.

5.39 A. True
  B. False
  C. True
  D. True
  E. False

Paediatric transplant recipients should all have prior immunization as giving any after transplant can cause problems from immunosuppression. Regular haemodialysis is not always necessary. It is, however, necessary to have an ultrasound of the major blood vessels to make certain that the blood vessels are all patent and that there are no congenital anomalies. A well-matched transplant kidney will of course help obtain prolonged graft and patient survival.

5.40 A. False
  B. False
  C. False
  D. True
  E. False

Perfusion with a cold iso-osmolar solution preserves the millieu interior of a transplant kidney and will allow preservation in surrounding ice for a prolonged period. While machine preservation is practised by some surgeons, it is not essential. Any warm solution will increase the warm ischaemia time and decrease graft survival.

5.41 A. True
   B. True
   C. True
   D. True
   E. False

All patients in the end stage of renal failure should have electrolyte studies as well as renal function tests. As they are often prone to atherosclerotic ischaemic heart disease an ECG and CXR constitute baseline investigations. In the elderly, and where cardiac function is suspect on clinical grounds, the opinion of a cardiologist must be sought. Not everyone however requires a coronary angiogram, though echocardiograms are proving a useful non-invasive alternative.

5.42 A. True
   B. False
   C. False
   D. False
   E. True

A good arterial blood pressure and a CVP are crucial to good perfusion of the kidney. It is therefore essential that the anaesthetic techniques include methods to preserve these parameters. While helpful, epidural anaesthesia is not crucial to management. In the same way antibiotic therapy is not necessary, and immunosuppression is usually given prior to anaesthetic induction.

5.43 A. True
   B. False
   C. False
   D. True
   E. True

Although peritoneal dialysis is approximately one-eighth as efficient as haemodialysis in altering blood solute composition and one-fourth as efficient in terms of fluid removal, it can be carried out over 24 h, unlike haemodialysis which is usually for a maximum of 4 h a day. Hence on a daily basis the efficacy is not markedly different. PD is ideal for home use as patients can manage their dialysis independently, and preferred in infants and young children as it avoids repeated needling and allows ambulation. The gentler fluid shifts in PD as opposed to HD are likely to impose less strain on patients with poor cardiovascular function. Adhesions prevent safe insertion of PD catheters and compromise dialysate exchange and drainage.

5.44 A. True
   B. True
   C. False
   D. True
   E. False

There are no absolute contraindications to dialysis and the decision to treat is based on an ethical assessment of quality of life considerations. Age in itself is not a contraindication as many elderly patients are physiologically equivalent to younger persons. Hepatitis C is not a contraindication, though universal precautions against spread of infection need to be taken.

5.45 A. True
   B. True
   C. True
   D. True
   E. True

All of these conditions have dialysis as a valid intervention at some stage in their management protocol.

5.46 A. True
 B. True
 C. True
 D. True
 E. False

Congestive cardiac failure may be precipitated in patients with compromised cardiac function, as a result of increased cardiac output, especially in the upper arm or femoral fistulae. Infections are rare, but usually staphylococcal when they do occur.

5.47 A. True
 B. False
 C. True
 D. False
 E. True

Smaller molecular weight solutes diffuse more rapidly across a permeable membrane. The greater the hydrostatic pressure across a membrane, the greater the extent of ultrafiltration.

5.48 A. True
 B. True
 C. True
 D. True
 E. False

5.49 A. True
 B. False
 C. True
 D. True
 E. False

Dose-related renal arteriolar vasoconstiction, interstitial fibrosis and thrombotic microvascular disease are all caused by cyclosporin. Cyclosporin inhibits the production of vasodilatory nitric oxide by the endothelial cells.

5.50 **A.** True
B. False
C. True
D. False
E. True

Azathioprine can cause bone-marrow suppression and leucopenia, thrombocytopenia and macrocytic anaemia as well as hepatotoxicity, susceptibility to neoplasia and infection, increased viral warts and interactions with allopurinol. Osteoporosis and cataracts are seen in glucocorticoid excess.

5.51 **A.** True
B. True
C. True
D. True
E. False

Cyclosporin can also cause hepatotoxicity, hypertension and lymphoid tumours.

5.52 **A.** True
B. False
C. True
D. True
E. False

OKT3 only reacts with human T-cells. It invariably causes a febrile reaction on the first administration and can precipitate a fulminant pulmonary oedema if the patient is not euvolaemic or close to dry weight.

5.53 **A.** True
B. False
C. True
D. True
E. True

If the pretransplant crossmatch is positive then a hyperacute rejection is inevitable. Though acute rejection is primarily cellular, it can rarely be the result of an antibody-mediated kind of necrotizing arteritis or vascular rejection.

5.54 A. True
   B. True
   C. False
   D. True
   E. True

The incidence of abdominal wall hernias in PD patients can be as high as 10%. They are prone to develop sclerosing peritonitis and consequent bowel obstruction. The incidence of diverticulosis is no higher, though patients of adult polycystic disease have an incidence of diverticular disease as high as 86% in some studies. Ischaemic bowel can be precipitated by a combination of underlying vascular disease and raised intra-abdominal pressure during PD. Complaints of low back pain are not infrequent.

5.55 A. True
   B. True
   C. True
   D. True
   E. False

5.56 A. True
   B. True
   C. True
   D. True
   E. True

Index